Valarie Dominamb

D1430955

Anorexia Nervosa
The Broken Circle

ANOREXIA NERVOSA
The Broken Circle

ANN ERICHSEN

with an introduction by
PETER DALLY
MB, FRCP, FRCPsych, DPM

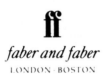

faber and faber
LONDON · BOSTON

First published in 1985
by Faber and Faber Limited
3 Queen Square, London WC1N 3AU

Filmset by Goodfellow & Egan Cambridge
Printed in Great Britain by
Thetford Press Limited
Thetford, Norfolk
All rights reserved

British Library Cataloguing in Publication Data

Erichsen, Ann
Anorexia nervosa : the broken circle
1. Anorexia nervosa—Patients—Biography
I. Title
616.85'2   RC552.A5
ISBN 0-571-13537-4

Contents

Acknowledgements

The quotations from T. S. Eliot's *Four Quartets* are from 'East Coker' and 'Little Gidding' and are included by permission of Faber and Faber, London, and Harcourt, Brace Jovanovich Inc., New York. (USA: Copyright 1943 by T. S. Eliot; renewed 1971 by Esme Valerie Eliot.)

The lines of Rainer Maria Rilke are taken from *An Unofficial Rilke*, selected, introduced and translated by Michael Hamburger. They are used by permission of the publishers, Anvil Press Poetry Limited, London SE10 8PX.

Author's Preface

My daughter had anorexia nervosa. There are thousands of other mothers who also have daughters with anorexia nervosa and are unable to find help and support. This book is for them and about them. When my daughter was first ill I read all the available books, both lay and medical, and found that although they were carefully and sensitively written to give a clear picture of the illness and of its possible length and outcome they were not helpful as far as daily living was concerned.

There seemed to be a genuine need for a book which would remove some of the mystery and misconception surrounding the illness and give mothers practical suggestions for coping with a distressing and difficult situation.

This book is not an intellectual *tour de force* or a medical textbook. It is an attempt to view anorexia nervosa from the inside, to put it into a wider perspective, to take an objective look at it from a subjective standpoint. It is based on the experiences not only of many mothers who have talked to me, often at the cost of considerable personal distress, but also of a cross-section of sufferers. Some of these have been ill for up to 25 years, some have recovered completely.

Every anorectic is an individual but there are a number of common factors, some of which occur in every case. Mothers were anxious that they or their daughters might be recognised but no case histories are used as my intention was always to make a composite picture of the illness from the mothers' point of view. I would not have asked them to talk to me on any other basis. It has been painful to write and some people may find parts of it painful and uncomfortable to read. Mothers will realise that any criticisms are also likely to apply to *me*, although this is intended to be neither an attack nor an apology.

Inevitably questions are aired about a number of issues which affect us all – anorexia nervosa and its accompanying chaos represent many of the problems of modern life. Why do people find it difficult to communicate with one another? Do we expect too much of our children, ourselves, our families, our doctors? Are the difficulties which parents experience with the medical profession due to incompetence and the lack of sensible advice or to parents, particularly mothers, being unwilling or unable to listen carefully to advice which they are given?

Are the difficulties between parents and psychiatrists due to the fear of mental illness, or has the psychiatric assertion that the refusal to accept psychiatric help is irrefutable evidence of a disorder of the psyche simply rebounded upon them? Is the damage to the families of anorectics due to ignorance and lack of information rather than to an intrinsic weakness in malfunctioning families? Is anorexia nervosa at least partly caused through brainwashing by the media and by the need of a capitalist society to make increasingly large profits, regardless of damage to the consumer, in order to perpetuate itself? Or is it the result of a large number of mothers' increasing inability to relate to, and accept, current attitudes towards adolescence and the female condition?

This book is also for me. I had hoped by writing and researching it to find answers to my daughter's problems and perhaps to be able to shift some of the inevitable burden of guilt and bitter regret on to someone else. This I have not been able to do but by reading widely and by having the privilege of talking to so many intelligent, articulate and caring mothers, patients and professionals I have been able to understand and accept my own responsibility and to realise its limits.

I have been luckier than most other mothers in that I have always been dealt with kindly and gently by all the doctors with whom I have come into contact, from our own GP to my daughter's consultant. Even so, there have been moments when I have been resentful and rebellious, hypersensitive to my own feelings, impervious to other people's, thinking only of my despair at seeing my daughter so ill and unhappy. Like many other mothers, I have sometimes failed to listen carefully to, and absorb, advice, often because my ignorance of the condition made the advice given seem irrelevant or unacceptable.

I have been criticised for writing this book. Naturally, there have been times when I have wondered whether it would damage my daughter, whether it was absorbing more time than could or should be spared from her sister and brother. It gave me many opportunities of discussing various aspects of anorexia nervosa with her unemotionally and helped me to know what to do when she was ready to get better.

All the mothers I interviewed wanted to 'do something to help' but did not know how to go about it. I am deeply grateful to them all, and to the past and present sufferers who talked to me, for bravely and generously sharing their experiences with me. All of them hoped that this book will give constructive help to other women suspecting, living with and trying to defeat anorexia nervosa.

I would also like to thank all the professionals who patiently discussed anorexia nervosa with me, my family and friends for their unfailing support and interest, and Miss Patricia Downie of Faber and Faber for her sound advice.

Finally, I want to thank Doctor Peter Dally of the Westminster Hospital for his infinite kindness and patience, his depth of knowledge and understanding, and for the bracing encouragement and practical help without which this book could never have been written.

I have referred throughout the book to sufferers from anorexia nervosa as female, i.e. as a girl/girls, or as a daughter/daughters. This was partly because it allowed the text to flow more easily, and partly because most of the mothers to whom I talked had daughters rather than sons with anorexia nervosa.

At least 1 in 20 anorectics are male, and while any general comments on the background and management of anorexia nervosa are relevant there are differences due to sex which make it essential for parents whose son develops anorexia nervosa to seek specialised help.

SPECIALIST TERMS

I have tried to avoid the use of psychiatric jargon but certain terms cannot be replaced – the three most commonly encountered are as follows:

abreaction   The removal by revival and expression of the emotion associated with an event which has been buried in a person's mind in such a way as to inhibit development and mental health.

'*acting out*'   The description sometimes given to the antisocial or disruptive behaviour of people who are either unable to express their fears and worries verbally or who feel that no one would have the time or wish to listen to them if they were to attempt to do so.

individuation   Described by Jung as one of the tasks of middle age, it is also one of the tasks of puberty. It is the process by which people realise that they have, and are entitled to have, their own identity and personality, regardless of the effect it may have on the self-interest or needs of those with whom they live.

Introduction
by PETER DALLY MB, FRCP, FRCPsych, DPM

There are few illnesses which cause so much distress and
derangement within the sufferer's family as anorexia nervosa.
A painful, chronic, or fatal illness in a child or parent
obviously upsets everyone. But at least there is a clearcut
problem which can be understood, accepted and adapted to
more or less. Even a psychiatric disorder such as depression
or agoraphobia can be accommodated within the family. But
for the relatives of a girl who develops anorexia nervosa
there is fury, pity, guilt, despair, every kind of feeling except
that of happiness and contentment. For here, in the heart of
the family, is a child who refuses to eat the family's food,
who may even refuse to eat with them, who is suddenly an
intrusive irritant, destroying the centre of family life. The
parents are outraged, their peace of mind destroyed by their
daughter's incomprehensible and intransigent behaviour.
Siblings are upset by the continual rows at mealtimes, jealous
of the attention their sister attracts. No one can understand,
no one can accept what is happening.

They have almost certainly read or heard of anorexia
nervosa, but that such a condition can affect one of their
children has rarely occurred to parents. They feel angry,
ashamed and, sooner or later, helpless. They seek the aid of
their doctor, expecting him to relieve their distress and solve
the problem as though it were a common cold. When he fails
to give instant relief their rage may turn against him. He

becomes the scapegoat. If only he had done this or that the matter would have been quickly resolved. They seek other opinions and not only medical ones. For where specific treatment of a condition is lacking, quacks and practitioners of alternative medicine thrive. The more parents rush from pillar to post, the worse the problem becomes. Until they can stop the merry-go-round, step on to firm ground and look long and hard and honestly at the problem and themselves, there is little chance of any improvement. This is none too easy, but it is the turning point. For anorexia nervosa always involves other people as well as the sufferer herself. And since the vast majority of patients are adolescent, these other people are almost invariably her close family. Even if, at the beginning of the trouble, the family seems blissfully united, sooner rather than later it will come under increasing strain and ominous cracks will appear.

Of course, anorexia nervosa is not *just* due to family problems. It is essentially a psychosomatic disorder, a complex interdependent mind/body interaction, involving numerous factors, many of which are here discussed.

Cultural influences are strong in many illnesses but particularly psychiatric, affecting not only the incidence but also the symptomatology. To take one example, in their tribal culture Africans show a very low incidence of neurosis, but once they become urbanised and subjected to European cultural patterns the incidence of neurosis rises rapidly to European levels. Our own society today emphasises slimness in women. Hilde Bruch has speculated that 'the enormous emphasis fashion places on slimness' may be responsible for the increase in anorexia nervosa during the past 15–20 years. Most adolescents diet at some time, partly to identify with their peers, and largely to emphasise that they are shedding their puppy fat, changing from schoolgirls to sophisticated young women. In reality, few need to diet seriously. But even when a girl is overweight and can reasonably lose a stone or more, something more than just a wish to diet and lose weight grows in the mind of the girl with anorexia nervosa. She becomes terrified of the strength of her appetite, fearful that she may lose control of it, and so put on a huge amount of weight and become fat. She inhibits, by superhuman efforts, her hunger and appetite. Her weight falls, often to dangerous levels. Friends and relatives fear the worst if she continues unabated. But the girl herself has no wish to die. Rather, anorexia nervosa expresses her doubts and confusion, her uncertainty about how to behave, her fears of failure, of not coming up to her own high expectations. As a sense of failure grows, so she feels increasingly 'empty', worthless, and unlovable.

It is understandable for these girls to turn to the one thing they can control, their size. Slimness is goodness, so why not diet and lose weight? If they control their appetite they can achieve perfection. No longer will they let their bodies run riot and grow and change shape. They will exert complete control over their intake of food and weight. Fat bottoms, hips and thighs will disappear. They will achieve the *perfect* shape, the beauty of perfection.

But the nagging fear that they are imperfect remains; sooner or later they may lose control and become fat. Beneath their apparent lack of concern, terror is never far away.

Anorexia nervosa began to increase in the 1950s and reached a peak in the late 1970s. The vast number of victims are intelligent and attractive adolescent girls, from middle-class families. It may now have started to decline among this group of patients (at the same time starting to appear increasingly among older, often married women). How can one explain this phenomenal epidemic? Ann Erichsen has pointed to an important factor, the changes that have occurred in the lives of women over the past 30 years or so, not least the increased opportunities for education and careers, and the widespread change in sexual habits and mores. Many mothers of anorexic daughters look with some envy at the academic opportunities which now exist, which were not available to their generation. But if they missed out themselves they can at least ensure that their intelligent daughters are able to take full advantage of these opportunities. Considerable financial sacrifice may be made in sending a daughter to a private school, an aspect all too apparent to the girl. No matter that her parents repeatedly tell her that they are not ambitious for her to do well and only want her to be happy; the girl knows that this is not strictly true. Her own internal voices tell her that she must be successful to please her parents. Inevitably she trembles when she faces important exams. However much her teachers assure her that she is certain to pass with flying colours, and her parents try to make light of the exam, the voice of conscience insists that she has not worked sufficiently hard to achieve everything her parents expect of her and, more important, that she expects of herself. She will fail.

She determines to work more intensively and to keep her thoughts entirely centered on her studies. But it is difficult for a healthy 15 or 16-year-old girl to keep her mind entirely on her work and off sex. Her friends talk of little else, some are on the Pill, one may have had an abortion. Newspapers and magazines, television, even the compulsory D. H. Lawrence novel she has to read for A-level English, fire her fantasies. She knows that her mother is right, that sex and school work are incompatible. There is plenty of time for sex after she has finished her exams. She must suppress her increasingly troublesome feelings and thoughts. She must gain control over her emotions and her body. And lo and behold, she does gain control of her sexual feelings as she diets and loses weight. The thinner she is, the less troublesome is sexuality. Thinness is safe and good. Yet reality is not entirely lost. One part of her is pleased, but another is horrified. She is aware that she looks awful at 31kg (68lb), even though she delights to be this weight, feeling to be in control of her appetite. She feels attractive within herself, however unattractive she may appear to others.

18

Food allergies, dietary eccentricities, other cases of anorexia nervosa, often feature in the history of patients' families. Sisters are most obviously affected by their sibling's behaviour. Anorexia nervosa is an 'infectious' condition. Even in institutions wider than the family, for instance a girls' boarding school, anorexia nervosa can spread wildly from an anorexic girl to her fellows. This was particularly so 10 or 15 years ago. Headmistresses dreaded the onset of a serious case and usually ordered the victim home, knowing that unless they did so susceptible girls would begin to succumb.

Mothers and maternal grandmothers of patients may show anorexia nervosa-like behaviour or even frank anorexia nervosa, although rarely prolonged and intense. An aunt, on the other hand, or an older cousin, is not uncommonly found to have chronic anorexia nervosa. It is extremely rare for a brother to be affected. The incidence of anorexia nervosa in males is about 20 times less than that among women of comparable age.

Is it likely that anorexia nervosa can be accounted for by genetic factors? No one, of course, will suggest that anorexia nervosa is inherited *per se*. But it may be that a particular kind of genetic constitution must be present in order for specific environmental factors to produce their effects. To use a gardening metaphor, just as rhododendrons will flourish only in acid soil free of lime, perhaps anorexia nervosa will only develop when the structure of the nervous system is a suitable one. There is some evidence for this. Depressive illness, including manic depression, and alcoholism, where genetic influences play an important role, are not uncommon in the relatives of anorexic patients. A predisposition may be inherited which, depending on circumstances and experiences, will manifest itself later in one of several ways. In this context it may be significant that depression frequently develops at some stage, and that alcoholism is often a complication in established anorexia nervosa, particularly in those patients who progress from controlling their weight by strict dieting alone to using vomiting and laxative abuse.

It is clear that there is never *one* cause of anorexia nervosa. Many factors are concerned in the development and continuation of the condition, and they interact subtly. In any one patient the importance of this or that factor will vary, but ultimately, when pressure is sufficiently high, anorexia nervosa develops. It is this variation in causal forces which creates confusion among researchers, for patients may seem to have very different profiles and backgrounds; one was a fat child, another comes from an unhappy home, has a professionally successful mother, had to change schools frequently, and so on. No one patient can be understood unless the detailed circumstances of her life and family are fully known. Even then we must recognise that many of the factors which seem important can be found in adolescents who never develop anorexia nervosa. They are protected by their outgoing personalities, by 'strengths' provided within their families – a close relationship with an older sibling, a grandmother or other relative, or by friends. A case of anorexia nervosa can only begin to be comprehended if all features, both negative and positive, however ill-defined, are recognised.

The precipitating event which starts anorexia nervosa is merely the trigger which fires the loaded gun. It is often a looming event like O- and A-level examinations which activate the girl's fear of failure. It may be a separation from or loss of someone on whom she depends; sometimes a death, but more often the absence of a trusted person in whom she could confide. Frequently it is some change which upsets family balance and stability; father losing his job, moving home, a financial crisis, illness of a close relative. Sexual traumas, family scandals, a sister's abortion or shotgun marriage are uncommon precipitants. By contrast, upsetting sexual happenings are common precipitating events when anorexia nervosa starts in the 20s or later. A physical illness, with the possible exception of glandular fever, is unusual.

Once anorexia nervosa starts it is generally unstoppable for a time at least. Mild cases recover within six or nine months with little or no treatment or disruption of family life. These form the vast majority of cases. But some continue. Weight loss gathers momentum and destructive power. These are the patients who are seen by psychiatrists, who sometimes die, whose development so often comes to a halt, whose families suffer and may be irretrievably reft.

If doctors understand the condition, and the reasons why a girl needs to become emaciated, why cannot she and her family be helped more and sooner? Ann Erichsen describes the feelings of parents and patients well, their frustrations, anxiety, and increasing bewilderment and helplessness. And, more important, she discusses what happens to the family and how the family itself, especially the mother, can best tackle the problem. She criticises the medical profession, not least psychiatrists, for what often seems to be arrogant insensitive behaviour, the attitude of 'I know best'. But in truth a skirmish between psychiatrist and parents over an adolescent daughter with anorexia nervosa is almost inevitable. The psychiatrist is, after all, intruding into the family and its secrets. He is taking over partial responsibility for the child's care because the parents see themselves as having failed. He is seen to be taking their child from them, perhaps encouraging her to think and behave in ways of which they disapprove. He is certain to be seen by most parents as a threat. Only rarely, when tensions between mother and father are high, is he likely to be welcomed as a friend and guide by one or the other – rarely by both.

Psychiatrists are acclimatised to strong reactions from patients and relatives. They do not immediately react angrily to hostility. They look for the reasons, and in so doing expand their understanding of the patient's illness. They treat the angry querulous parent(s) sympathetically, attempt to lessen their fears, and help them come to terms with the problem.

A psychiatrist must always be honest and frank, although not naive. But above all he must make it plain to the patient and her family that he will not take sides. The patient must recognise that he is not an agent of her parents, for only then can she trust him. Parents must accept that his role is to help their daughter develop self-confidence so that she no longer needs to cling childlike to them, or assert herself in maladaptive neurotic ways through food and weight. His aim is to help her to grow up, not to grow away from her parents.

Most adolescent disorders, including anorexia nervosa, clear up spontaneously within a year. But some cases continue for many years and a few never resolve. Only if the factors which are responsible for perpetuating the condition are recognised is it possible to devise really effective long-term treatment. There are at least four issues.

The first is the degree of emaciation. Profound and widespread changes follow much loss of weight, particularly when body weight falls below 75 per cent of the ideal (usually calculated from insurance tables); for instance, a girl 165cm (65in) tall should be about 54kg (119lb) plus or minus 3.5kg (7lb); a 25 per cent loss brings her weight to 41kg (89lb) or lower. Output of hormones, particularly gonadal (sex) hormones, are then profoundly altered and perpetuate the amenorrhoea (cessation of menstruation) which has usually developed *with the onset* of serious dieting before much weight is lost. Most important of all are the psychological changes that accompany emaciation. The patient reverts to an earlier, more childlike way of thinking and feeling, and withdraws into herself. Mentally she comes to inhabit a fortress or prison, unhappy with conditions but unwilling to break out, terrified of the terrors that await her in the world outside. At low weight it is virtually impossible to develop the close empathy which is necessary for effective psychotherapy. Interesting discussions about her attitude to her weight and size, her sense of inner emptiness and ineffectiveness, the reasons why no one wants to be friendly towards her, are all possible, but they remain on an intellectual level and there is no accompanying release of feeling, no flow of warmth between therapist and patient. Psychotherapy can achieve little at low weight, apart from offering simple support. There is no likelihood of progress until the girl's weight returns to at least 80 per cent of her ideal weight, or previous weight if that was reasonable. Because of this it is essential to concentrate initially on regaining weight, and to do this it is often necessary to admit the girl to hospital. It is unusual for the girl to regain much weight while living at home, unless she has a mother as detached and strong as the author, and she can only achieve this after long tribulations.

Many parents regard their daughter's treatment in hospital, at least the initial part, as barbaric. They are not permitted to visit until the girl has regained an agreed amount of weight, and she herself is not allowed up to the toilet or bathroom until she reaches specified weight targets. Some hospitals insist on putting the girl into a bare single room, but this is really not necessary. Ann Erichsen criticises, rightly, the all too frequent lack of communication between parents and staff, which results in parents failing to understand what is really happening to their daughter and why. No wonder treatment often seems crude and cruel to them and raises doubts about the whole procedure. Since anorexia nervosa is all about the patient's inability to communicate and express feelings, it is curious that doctors and nurses do not lean over backwards to explain their plan of treatment and its rationale in detail to parents.

It is striking how the girl's psychosomatic health and vitality improve as her weight returns to a reasonable level. The intellectual protective wall cracks and falls, and she begins to show emotional warmth. Fear of increasing her size lessens and important issues can now be discussed in a meaningful way. She can at last begin to face her real problems and progress.

The second factor is the matter of the girl's lack of self-confidence, the chaotic state of her psyche. A large part of her is still a child, terrified of losing her parents' love and support. The need to please them is paramount. Anything she sets out to do is for their sake rather than because she wants to succeed or achieve something for herself. Her own self, the young woman she now is, is not allowed to emerge. Rebellious thoughts and urges that conflict with the standards and morals of her parents are suppressed. Emerging sexual needs are sublimated into work. Religious and political views are kept in line with those of her parents. Anger, which has seethed below the surface for so long, is utilised to strengthen the anorexic resistance to eating, and thereby kept out of sight.

All these so far unacceptable emotions and thoughts must be allowed to come into the open, and be recognised by the girl – or rather young woman – as part of herself. She is no longer totally dependent on her parents. She has to break with them in lots of ways if she is to express her own identity. Only when she has done this can she then move into a new and more adult relationship with them, where she can feel loved for her own sake and not for what she achieves or how she behaves.

This is where psychotherapy has such an important part to play once the girl has regained weight. She cannot talk about her deep feelings and fears with her parents or even her friends. She distrusts herself too much to confide fully in any of them. But a doctor or psychiatrist is different. He (or she) is not involved with her or her family emotionally. He is detached and his interest in her must mean that she is not wholly bad and beyond hope of recovery. He becomes a person she can trust and look upon as a kindly parent figure. She may resist at first, but before long she looks forward to seeing him. She thinks about him, as well as the topics they discuss. In a youthful adolescent sense he becomes her hero, someone around whom she can weave fairy tale fantasies. This is a somewhat crude description of *transference*, the

24

transference on to the psychiatrist, or whoever is in a comparable role, of the feelings a patient had as a child for his or her parents. Because he is perceived as good and loving, the patient feels secure enough to reveal herself, to accept her adult status, with everything that goes with that role. She may literally fall in love for a time, which does no harm, and much good, provided the psychiatrist is competent. In time the girl is gradually weaned on to more realistic and normal relationships.

Ann Erichsen asks whether the creation of transference is 'morally sound' or the 'ultimate dirty trick'. It can only be immoral if the psychiatrist takes advantage of it for his own gain, or is unwilling to complete what he started. It is a powerful non-specific force, which all clinicians, not just psychiatrists, use in some measure. Even the effects of a pill, good and bad, are strongly influenced by whether or not a patient likes or dislikes the doctor prescribing the drug. However, it is not difficult to see that a parent may over-react to a daughter's positive transference. Father may see the psychiatrist as a rival for his daughter's affections. Mother may herself be attracted and wish to step into her daughter's shoes. Family life can be something of a whirlwind so far as psychiatry is concerned!

The third perpetuating factor of importance is the absence of a social life. Many of the more severely affected patients are ill for at least three or four years, and during this time they are too timid and withdrawn to mix with former friends, or to form new ones. In consequence they find themselves socially isolated as they begin to near the final stages of recovery. Not only are they without friends but they also lack social knowhow; they do not know how they should react in social situations. They continue to shy away from contact with their peers for fear of inappropriate behaviour, of making fools of themselves, and particularly so where young men are concerned. Adolescence, especially the latter half and the early 20s, is a time when social confidence is learnt and developed and permanent deep friendships are made. The gap that exists in the experience of an anorexia patient is a serious one which may hold her back indefinitely from taking the final step to recovery and freedom.

To help her overcome this the patient is encouraged to join one or more small therapeutic groups (of six or seven young-ish people of both sexes). This starts once she has regained weight. The group meets once or twice a week and discusses a range of subjects which concern or touch upon the group members' problems. The girl gains confidence through being able to discuss not only her own but the problems of others. She is able to recognise that her fears and difficulties are not unique, and she gains from learning how other people cope with their anxieties. Inevitably there are emotional inter-actions within the group, and the girl has to cope not only with her own feelings but with those of her fellows, ranging from angry outbursts to affectionate approval. In addition, she is often included in a special social skills group. Here, encounters and situations which appear frightening are acted out, with members of the group playing appropriate roles, under the direction of an occupational therapist; for in-stance, meeting a young man at a party, an interview for a job, buying a dress and trying it on before sales assistants, taking part in a lunch party, visiting a disco with friends, and so on. As self-confidence is gained, play-acting gives way to reality. The girl is encouraged to contact and take up with her old friends, or to join a club, to renew her wardrobe, and generally move back into society. Gradually, if all goes well, she begins to compete with and enjoy the company of her friends. She is now able to eat with them without feeling greedy, and no longer has to compare her intake of food with theirs. She may continue for many months to think obsess-ively about food and weight, but her behaviour will no longer be dominated by such thoughts. With time their intensity progressively lessens.

The fourth factor concerns the girl's family. The adolescent girl with anorexia nervosa has become trapped within her family, unable to express openly her real feelings and aspirations, forced ultimately to use eating and weight as a means of communicating her needs. A 'double-bind' situation arises. The girl says one thing, 'I am happy and content with my parents', yet contradicts herself by refusing to eat normal family meals or even to eat at all with her parents, which translated means, 'I am angry and unhappy but I don't dare tell you to your face.' Some of the problems and tensions within the family which have contributed to the girl's anorexia nervosa are mentioned above. Ann Erichsen discusses them in detail and with insight. She describes some of the difficulties of her own marriage which eventually ended in divorce. She believes, with some truth, that 'a girl whose parents are happily married, and (adult like) are sympathetic to each other's values and points of view, is unlikely to develop anorexia nervosa.' That does not mean to say that *every* girl with anorexia nervosa comes from an unhappy family liable to disrupt at any moment. Other factors may have much stronger effects. But if a family is reasonably well-adjusted, and able quickly to recognise what may have gone wrong from their daughter's point of view, anorexia nervosa is unlikely to persist for long. When anorexia nervosa does continue for years it is usually because the factors responsible for the condition in the beginning are still present. When the girl regains weight in hospital, only to lose it as soon as she returns home, it is probable that family tensions remain unchanged. Conflicts in the families of anorexia nervosa parents are often concealed from outsiders, and even when mentioned they are likely to be minimised. The anorexic daughter is often reluctant to disclose family problems, especially if she feels they are largely her fault or that she must help to keep her parents together whatever the cost to her, which may include indefinite continuation of a 'sick role'.

It is essential for the psychiatrist to explore family relationships in these cases, to bring them to the surface so that they may be examined and, if possible, transmogrified. Occasionally this can contribute to the break-up of a marriage. Psychiatrists are frequently blamed and vilified for such happenings. But no psychiatrist *wishes* to see the end of the family. Divorce is a tragedy for everyone. The emotional security and development of children are threatened, and one or both parents may be seriously depressed for years. But a miserable marriage, riddled with conflict openly expressed or continuously bypassed, is even worse in its effects on children and on the parents. A family environment of persistent bitterness and despair is highly destructive, especially to the development of children and the growth of their 'identity'.

Until something is done to help the family resolve its difficulties, the girl with anorexia nervosa will continue to relapse, however much she is supported. *Family therapy* is the means by which psychiatrists try to treat the family, to help its members modify their relationships with one another and the whole, so that a happier, more open and honest family life may develop. In some cases everyone attends the meeting – with the psychiatrist and/or another staff member. But not everyone is always willing to come, and the group is often made up only of one or both parents and the patient. There is no point in forcing an unwilling sibling or parent to come. Meetings are usually held at weekly intervals at first. Some psychiatrists prefer to meet at the patient's home, and even to conduct the meeting over a meal, but I feel there is little to gain from this.

The anorexic daughter is encouraged to express her feelings about the family, to criticise in adult style their attitudes and behaviour towards her, and say why she feels resentful. During such sessions strong emotions often appear, and the characteristic rigid control that formerly existed in the family is, hopefully, replaced by increasingly adaptable attitudes.

When the patient, having regained weight, goes home from hospital – at first for a weekend – her increased self-confidence, with understanding and help from her parents, should allow her to speak her mind more freely and honestly. If she cannot she will, inevitably, fall back on indirect communication again and lose weight. Loss of weight at this stage is not a cause for stricture, but an indication that what is still preventing the girl from expressing herself openly at home must be discussed, not only with the girl herself but also in the family therapy meetings. Sooner or later, if all goes well, the patient will feel confident enough to speak out her mind and eat comparatively normally, and resume a more normal outgoing life.

Treatment is always complex. There is no one method. All aspects of the girl's problem need to be tackled. A therapist should never give up. Every patient is, in theory at least, fully recoverable. But parents, as well as therapists, may despair, seek short cuts, demand a change of doctors, look for magic, anything but face painful reality. It takes courage and insight on the part of a parent to ensure that a daughter recovers. Ann Erichsen is such a one. The more she recognised that the anorexia nervosa of her daughter reflected what was happening within the family, the greater her determination to treat the problem as a *whole*, to accept her responsibility. It is impossible for anorexia nervosa to exist under such conditions. Ann Erichsen's description of her experience – her own and that gleaned from the many mothers of patients she has interviewed – and advice on what to expect and do if a child develops anorexia nervosa should be read by everyone who encounters this terrifying condition.

1

Anorexia Nervosa

You never know yourself till you know more than your
body. . . . In the knowledge of your powers, inclinations,
principles, the knowledge of yourself chiefly consisteth.

Thomas Traherne, *Centuries of Meditations.*

Throughout over a century of changing views and treatments
of patients with anorexia nervosa, medical attitudes to their
mothers have remained constant. 'Experience shows repeatedly, though it is not always easy to understand the reason,
that it is the mothers whose influence is so deleterious, who
will hear no argument and will only yield in general to the
last extremity,' wrote Charcot in 1889. This opinion is still
held today.

Most mothers are soon made aware of this and would
welcome more direct criticism, realistic advice, clearer explanation of the illness and the usual surrounding circumstances. They are not afraid to face the situation or to accept
any necessary or possible changes provided they know what
is required of them and what others have found helpful.
Anorexia nervosa is surrounded by confusion and ignorance,
innuendo and presupposition. Mothers feel lost and helpless,
floundering in deep waters with no hope of rescue.

Looking after a daughter or son with anorexia nervosa has
the same psychological effect on the mother as being slapped
across the face several times a day for a considerable period
of time. There is the same loss of equilibrium, the same slight
nausea and fear and the same overpowering need to hold on

to her own identity, since the failure to do so would undermine her completely. It is a way of life almost impossible to describe and only made comprehensible by personal experience.

Anorexia nervosa is a complicated and difficult illness. Many mothers are surprised it is still receiving the same treatment as it did over a hundred years ago. The incidence is rising but the outlook for patients is not improving. Many families, while grateful for emergency medical intervention, still find their greatest hope and help lie in the age-old remedies of time and prayer.

Anorexia nervosa occurs when a certain type of person is faced with a combination of problems at a particularly vulnerable stage in their development. The vulnerability has often been exacerbated by a fairly acute illness such as glandular fever, meningitis, rheumatic fever or acute measles. The usual preconditions and common factors include: ambition, despair, a paralysing sense of ineffectiveness, social mobility, psychosomatic illnesses of various kinds earlier in childhood, jealousy, insecurity, fear, restriction and repression, denial of marital and family problems, sexual inhibitions, unhappiness, despondency, anger, panic, frustration, aimlessness, depression, tension of various kinds, stress, distorted control, hysteria and obsessiveness.

What is anorexia nervosa? What is its purpose and its rewards? Is it produced by the self-defeating thrills of vicarious living or by the anger of passive tension? Is it decadence or defence, defiance or despair? Is it anarchy or anguish? Is it a cry for help or a throwing down of the gauntlet? Is it catharsis or catalyst, reaction or revenge? Are its rituals an attempt to re-create a rigid structure which has been rejected by the patient's parents? Is it the setting up of an alternative one-person government to control a family unable to function efficiently because it is impervious to change? Is it a death wish, a longing for more excitement, or a prolonged fit of the vapours?

Medical labels vary from a functional nervous disorder to a psychosomatic illness and an adolescent neurosis. It is also described as a psychologically adaptive stance operating within biological mechanisms, a maturational crisis, a collection of different psychiatric syndromes under one name, a defence against prostitution, a retreat from incest, an ascetic stance stemming from a profound spiritual vacuum, an unresolved conflict of the mother being acted out by her daughter, an escape route for the spoilt rich brat, the result of pathological symbiotic hold, a chronic food allergy, a biochemical imbalance, a hypothalamic dysfunction, a family problem with the anorectic acting the role of scapegoat, a condition arising from a failed perfectionist using her body as a scapegoat, an extreme example of the notorious perversity of young girls.

It is also seen as illustrating the seeking and regulation of pleasure, the pride in self-control, which manifest in excessive dieting and in an unrealistic ideal of fitness. The anorectic's striving for thinness is seen as part of the current pursuit of perfection, control and mastery over body and mind and of the representation of these in the ego ideal. This pursuit also exists in swimmers, dancers, creative artists and other perfectionists.

Modern pressure on women to be slim and therefore attractive, advocated by an enormous number of books and magazine articles, is frequently blamed for the onset of the illness. A great number of females try to lose weight and a small proportion of these go on to develop anorexia nervosa. However, were it the fashion to be plump, the girls who develop anorexia nervosa would not spend their time eating cream buns and gorging as many calories per day as possible. The thinness is usually symbolic of far greater needs and conflicts than the pressures of fashion would produce.

Anorexia nervosa is popularly regarded as self-induced and so under the patient's control – she can recover exactly when she chooses to do so. There is no understanding, quite naturally, of the difficult lives these girls have and of the distress and damage to their families. No one who has even the smallest experience of anorexia nervosa can possibly imagine for one moment that the apparent benefits of extra attention and care compensate in any way for the unhappiness, physical discomfort and fatigue, panic, guilt, and social difficulties which patients endure. Nearly all are subjected in some degree to emotional, mental and sometimes physical battering both from their own families and from outsiders. A hunger strike is well known to arouse strong and hostile reactions. Anorexia nervosa has the same effect.

Anorexia nervosa is to some extent a maturational crisis, a problem of normal growth. Psychiatrists maintain that this only manifests when background problems and pressures trigger off anorexia nervosa. There used to be a perfectly acceptable condition known as 'outgrowing your strength'. In our present high-drive society even temporary frailty is unacceptable. The more fragile the foundations of any society the less it is able to tolerate weakness in its individual members.

Anorexia nervosa is sometimes seen as a by-product of capitalism, the flip side of affluence, or as a neurotic reaction to the levelling effect of bureaucracy and socialism, a desperate need to be mentally and physically free, coupled with an agonising inability to be either.

For many sufferers the future is a void. Mothers have to face the fact of having a daughter who is not only physically starving but who seems to be emotionally and spiritually without hope of nourishment. This is for some women the greatest anguish of all.

In order to understand anorexia nervosa it is necessary to look at its history and the social and economic changes which fostered it. Isolated cases have been well documented since the Middle Ages but it is principally a nineteenth-century illness, named 'anorexia nervosa' by Sir William Gull in 1874. It was as flourishing then as it is now and it is valid to place it in the social and economic setting where it belongs.

34

Its eruption in the 1860s must have been a reaction of some sort. Why? And to what?

It is easy to imagine anorexia nervosa as an example of nineteenth-century malaise – a pale and fragile girl, languishing romantically upon a sofa, summoning up just enough energy to ring for the maid, carefully looked after by her devoted family, united possibly for the first time by their mutual care and concern for their ailing daughter. Every little whim would have been catered for by her distraught mother, small delicacies provided, the siblings forced into a concern they may have felt to be unjustified, their own needs largely ignored and dismissed as irrelevant self-indulgence. She might have been visited by an adoring young man, whose visits would have exhausted nothing but her eyelashes. The truth was very different.

Death was a grim reality for many young people. Tuberculosis, whether psychogenic or not, was rampant, and scarlet fever, diphtheria and other infectious diseases fatal. So then, even more perhaps than now when we have vastly improved drugs and medical care, an apparently self-induced illness of such severity, a headlong flight from life, must have been particularly hard to understand.

The illness has quite rightly been viewed in many different ways and from many different angles, but always with an underlying theme of over-involvement between mother and daughter. The mother has been seen variously as neurotic, over-protective, over-possessive, maternally incompetent, withdrawn, vacillating, hysterical, depressed, dominant, dominating, domineering, rigid, frigid and even lesbian.

Anorexia nervosa is a complicated and little-understood illness and like all neuroses has to be looked at in the context both of the family which produces it and of the society which produced the family. The daughters of dedicated career women and rampant feminists develop it, as do those whose mothers are able to find fulfilment in the traditional domestic role within their own family and marriage.

35

Working mothers, whether they do so from choice or necessity, tend to have a strong enough sense of their own identity to foster that of their daughters. They are too physically exhausted and too mentally occupied to be over-protective and over-involved with their children. Against these advantages there is of course the plight of the latch-key child, often a distressed and distressing figure and on the increase. Some women are lucky and clever enough to find the right balance between domestic happiness – untramelled by frustration and resentment towards their husbands and children and the limits which their existence must inevitably impose upon a possibly pointless search for self-fulfilment – and the demands of a successful career.

There have been enormous changes in the female condition over the last 150 years. Marriage and traditional female occupations and virtues have undergone constant subtle changes. Theory has succeeded theory, leaving many mothers reeling under the psychological battering they receive from so-called experts, few of whom appear to have much if any personal practical experience of the problems to which they hope to provide answers. When instinct surrenders to infor-mation, unhappiness and difficulties tend to follow. Mothers of anorectics seem to have been particularly vulnerable to other people's advice.

The industrial revolution forced drastic changes upon a society which had previously been dependent upon agriculture for survival. During the nineteenth century the rapid move-ment of population into the towns led to communities and families being dispersed. A new middle class gradually emerged, lacking the confidence of tradition which provides a soothing sense of order and continuity and needing a structure within which to function. Its values became distorted, materialistic and artificial. Reality had to be excluded and so the ground was prepared in which neuroses could flourish.

The idealisation of childhood put children in a hopeless position by its demands that their behaviour should be better

36

than that of their parents, putting upon children the burden of a power they were unable to exercise. Boarding schools for girls provided opportunities for escape from the claustrophobic confinement of Victorian family life. An important function of equal rights feminism for the single woman was to fight for better educational facilities.

Many women in the last century preferred celibacy to the stagnation and restriction of contemporary marriage. Men could escape into military, civil service and commercial careers but their wives and sisters were largely restricted to the smaller sphere of musical evenings, embroidery, *Kirche, Küche, Kinder*, and good works.

Many girls were happy to fall into this undemanding existence, untroubled by the storm clouds of feminism swirling around their heads. Others fumed and fretted at the petty conventions and restrictions. These daughters were not naturally conformist, and could not and would not accept the apparently satisfactory future mapped out for them by their parents. Their fathers had often worked hard to improve their social and economic standing. Then, as now, the daughter was expected to continue this trend – in the last century by contracting a suitable and elevating marriage, and now, by performing well academically and socially.

Some girls were able to escape, but unfortunately girls with no income, gentler natures and possibly more domineering parents had only one way out – illness and hypochondria. Anorexia nervosa is a plea for autonomy, for self-determination, for freedom. It is an internal fight against external domination which uses the enormous power of self-destruction as its main weapon.

The deadening lack of self-confidence, the compulsion to always put others first and themselves last, to hide pain and feeling, the battering of their egos, began to establish a relentless grip on middle- and upper-class women. A high moral tone, bolstered by guilt, ensured that most women were protected and supported by their husbands and families. Anaesthetics began to be used in childbirth in 1847 and it is easy for an amateur to see this as having had dire effects on the mother/child relationship. It was part of a pattern of withdrawal from experience which fostered neurosis.

However, the increasing use of contraception and a wider understanding of the dangers of sexual repression and inhibition helped later to restore a more natural attitude to sexual needs and fulfilment within marriage. The female orgasm is popularly supposed to have disappeared overnight in Victorian England, to be fairly rapidly rediscovered with sighs of relief, notably by Sir Richard Burton. How a whole generation of women can seriously be supposed to have managed to conceal their response and pleasure from their husbands defies imagination. As the self-protective myth of the 'nice woman' gathered strength so did prostitution and the extra-marital passions so publicly enjoyed by Edward VII among many others.

Looking backward to previous generations of wives and mothers we see how our own lives have narrowed and changed. Until the last war most women had far more physical exercise than we do. They walked, rode or bicycled as a matter of course, motoring was a treat and pleasure, not the daily frustration it has now become. They were able to travel more slowly and more satisfyingly. They were not expected to be able to do so much so well. They did not feel it incumbent upon them, and nor did their husbands, to become Cordon Bleu cooks, expert dressmakers, home decorators, managing directors, enthusiastic gardeners, plumbers, happy and relaxed mothers of high-performing, well-adjusted children. They did not feel guilty if they took time to recover properly after the birth of each child.

Those who worked did not feel guilty if they employed other people to help with the domestic chores and were mercifully free of the compulsion to rush home and bash out their guilt on a lump of dough. They had a healthier diet,

38

processed foods beginning in the 1870s but not being used in quantity until an ever-increasing population and extensive housing development made home-grown food impossible for many.

They were not burdened by high academic expectations from their parents and a spinster daughter was seldom a source of embarrassment and conjecture. Celibacy did not have the slur of possible homosexuality which must have some bearing on the rising and early marriage rate, matched by the increasing divorce rate.

There was far better communication between people. They talked to each other more, found interest and amusement within themselves and their surroundings, used their wits and imaginations. A great deal of frustration was released in outpourings into diaries and in long and detailed letters. There was no television for the husband to slump in front of, semi-comatose and open mouthed, no loud canned music to deaden the adolescent senses and deafen the parents.

Mothers of anorectics mention the bad effects of television on their daughters. The physical violence and explicit sexual scenes can be disturbing to anyone sensitive and possibly inhibited. Far more serious is the way in which television aids and abets withdrawal. A mother whose daughter is watching television is able to have the comfortable feeling that she is happily occupied. She realises too late that she has been silently and imperceptibly disengaging from her family, and this at a stage when she has probably already largely withdrawn from her peers. The lack of conversation in so many families is a very sad reflection of an age in which people have too much leisure but not enough time.

Family groups tended to be larger with less clearly defined boundaries. The elderly stayed with or near their families, providing some sort of a lynch-pin for the younger members of the family and most importantly a sense of continuity, of acquired and transferable experience.

Many parents of teenage children today have never been

tried and tested as were their parents, their experiences have been too limited. The first generation who 'never had it so good' have never had it bad enough. They have never known the painful pleasures of contrast, of tragedy and farce, high adventure and low behaviour, joy and despair, acute and overwhelming relief within a wider setting than that of their immediate family. They have never been strengthened by meeting and defeating danger or had their resolve hardened by prolonged adversity. They have had too little demanded of them.

They find their authority and self-confidence diminished by their feelings of inadequacy and frustration at having had no real opportunity to prove themselves in other than the most mundane ways. Vicarious living is no substitute for life in the fullest sense for the many people who would rather be half dead than half alive.

Again and again anyone who believes in the concept of a self-regulating psyche has to see anorexia nervosa as an unconscious self-protective mechanism resulting from the sufferers' knowledge that they are not tough enough to be grown up, an attempt to create and conquer internally what life does not produce externally, to be able to face the future in a more demanding world than that in which they have been brought up. No blame can be attached to either parents or children who, like most other people, are forced by circumstance, instinct and necessity to adopt a mode of life which is socially acceptable and economically viable.

However, an excessive emphasis on convention and conformity undoubtedly characterises most families of anorectics to a point where individuality and initiative are unacceptable, threatening and stifled. Children with a strong and determined temperament, which is not overcome by the fear of the unknown typical of an anorectic, are able to deal with their parents' fears by either ignoring them completely or by taking refuge in rebellion and open resistance. They are the lucky ones.

Girls who develop anorexia nervosa are intelligent and perceptive, perfectly well aware of the demands being made of them and of the sacrifices in personal integrity these can entail. They have the appearance, background and temperament traditionally accorded to the revolutionary. They are idealistic, artistic, aesthetic, frequently unrealistic, at once using and despising the advantages of their ostensibly easy lives.

For some of them anorexia nervosa is internalised anarchy. There is no vehicle of revolt available to them, no organisation to join, no leader to follow and admire. They are too young and often too privileged to be attracted to militant feminism, its attitudes to marriage, morality and men are at once too narrow and too wide ranging to be relevant to them and their immediate hopes and needs. Nor do conventional politics attract them. Many are curiously apathetic to political issues.

Children are told far too often that they have such an easy life now, all amusements provided for them and all doors open. But adolescents are looking into a future in which nothing is certain and for which the easy life their parents have striven to give them is not an adequate preparation. Anorectics, being intelligent, perceptive people, can see all too clearly that hard-won academic success may be useless when it comes to finding a job in a time of ever-increasing unemployment.

Many of these girls have been processed towards success, but since the 1960s the rewards of continuing effort and sustained motivation have seemed pale and dreary compared to those of instant stardom. The Beatles were in the vanguard of this trend, proving that educational prowess was not necessary for enormous popular success, life was for living and enjoying without qualification and qualifications. Youth was on a winning streak, accepted values open to question and debate, marriage and the family subjected to change and criticism, the capitalist system of Western society noticeably on the decline.

Behaviour is said to change 20 years after attitudes, so the increase in adolescent neurosis and juvenile delinquency is due to some extent to the failure of parents to adapt and readjust to the less materialistic ambitions, less clearly defined aims of so many people and to the widening socialisation and state control which make individual success less valid and in some cases a definite handicap.

2

Symptoms

I must create a system or be enslaved by another Man's;
I will not Reason and Compare; my business is to Create.

William Blake, 'Jerusalem'

It is not always clear to parents that anorexia nervosa is not merely a state of mind, a figment of the imagination, but a serious illness with specific symptoms which make diagnosis possible.

These are:

1. Active refusal by the patient to eat enough to maintain a normal weight and/or determined sustained efforts to prevent ingested food from being absorbed. This is done by means of vomiting and of consuming large quantities of laxatives.
2. Loss of at least 10 per cent of previous body weight.
3. Amenorrhoea of at least three months' duration when menstruation has previously been regular. If menstruation has been irregular with gaps of two or more months, the period of amenorrhoea must be six months or more.
4. The patient's age of onset usually lies between 11 and 35 years. Atypical anorexia nervosa can occur at any time after this and, very rarely, before this.
5. There must be no sign of organic disease which might account for weight loss, serious affective disorder or schizophrenia.

6. The presence of at least two of the following; amenor-rhoea, lanugo (excessive fine body hair), bradycardia (slow pulse rate), periods of over-activity, episodes of bulimia (uncontrolled gorging of food), vomiting.

Mothers say with hindsight that the symptoms of anorexia nervosa are not noticed early enough because of the family's lack of experience. There are girls who stopped gaining weight at a critical stage rather than lost weight, so delaying puberty. Mothers generally felt that a dramatic change of personality marked the start of anorexia nervosa. This was most often noticed in conjunction with – or following within six months at the most – a change of school, moving house, other major change or following a severe illness. It manifested particularly in the O- or A-level year for girls under 18, and after an unhappy sexual encounter for girls over 18. At the time it was seen as a sign of teenage difficulty, or a foretaste of things to come, rather than as an indication of impending illness.

The bad temper and moodiness were usually accompanied by the beginning of the withdrawal process which at the time and in the circumstances was often a great relief to the rest of the family. The withdrawal is hard to detect as it is often masked by obsessive working. Hour upon hour of homework is done, six books referred to where one would do, repeated visits made to the library. The handwriting becomes obsessively small and neat. Careful attention is paid to every detail, drawings become minute and painstaking. The parents are delighted, feeling that at last their daughter is taking life seriously and making a real effort to work hard. It is, they think, an auspicious beginning for her future success.

Parents become aware that their daughter is beginning to set rigid routines and timetables to which the rest of the family are expected to adhere. Any deviation from these produces violent outbreaks of panic and anger so a consistent effort is made to stick to them. Expeditions with friends are scorned as timewasting and frivolous. Sense of humour, frequently in decline in adolescence, appears to have almost vanished.

The mother begins to feel extremely dispirited. The rest of the family react according to their own personalities, invariably producing further problems and difficulties involving disruptive behaviour of various kinds and sometimes altered and tiresome eating patterns with which the hapless mother has to cope.

She finds her daughter exercising frenetically, sometimes getting up hours before the rest of the household in order to have 'a good work-out'. The rest of the family are often woken by the sound of hectic exercises so that by breakfast time they are in a state varying from mild irritation to thoroughly bad temper. The days start on a bad note and are unlikely to improve as they go on.

The mother finds her daughter no longer walks at a normal pace but charges about at astonishing speed, rushing up and down stairs at any opportunity. She firmly denies fatigue, giving the impression that she is terrified to stop in case she can never start again. In spite of increasing emaciation she denies she is too thin. She is genuinely unable to see that this is so.

Mothers mention how miserably cold their daughters feel. As the illness progresses acrocyanosis is frequently present. This is dry, roughened skin, purple or dark red in colour, with a bluish tinge to the finger nails, extending from above the wrists to the tips of the fingers and from above the knees to the toes. They go to bed at exactly the same time every night, usually much earlier or much later than anyone else. Some girls sleep but insomnia is a problem for many. The retreat to the bedroom may be a way to escape from their families and constant pressure to eat. It is of course another opportunity to exercise rigorously, undisturbed by comment.

Many girls go to bed wearing jersey and bedsocks and with hot water bottles and electric blankets, even in summer.

They need blankets, duvets, eiderdowns in enormous quantities. During the day some are muffled in thick clothes and enormous baggy sweaters even in the hottest weather. Others are to be seen in the snow or bitter cold wearing thin shirts and skirts, without coats or warm covering, apparently impervious to the weather. The anorectic's appearance may be bizarre. The exhausted mother is helplessly furious in the face of what she sees as yet another attempt to emphasise her inadequacies.

Girls may be heavily made-up, trying to hide their pallor and their greenish-grey skin. Their haggard faces and sad and distant eyes render this pointless and ineffectual. It is an unmistakable indication of a need for attention and help.

Nearly every family with an anorectic daughter has experienced an appalling summer holiday. This is often the first time they see their daughter in a swimsuit and fully observe the extent of her emaciation. This leads to devastating rows between the anorectic daughter and her horrified and angry parents.

The dieting may be dramatic and obvious with rapid weight loss, it may be a continuation of a chronic decline since childhood, it may fluctuate. Most commonly a girl drifts into dieting slowly so that no alarm is caused. It is accepted at first, especially if a girl is overweight. It may be months before her determination hardens and her family begin to be aware of danger.

The dieting usually begins some time after the initial withdrawal and by then the illness is well under way. Carbohydrates are gradually excluded from the diet, food is slipped surreptitiously into a napkin or pocket, then flushed down the lavatory or waste disposer or put into the dustbin. The dog puts on weight.

So many people diet and are weight conscious that dieting behaviour is not initially thought to be unusual or sinister. What is unusual and ominous is a sudden obsessive interest in food and in feeding and cooking for other people. Hours are spent making cakes and sweets, bazaars and school sales are well catered for, friends are supplied with food.

The mother is angry to find her kitchen littered with mixing bowls and saucepans, seldom washed or put away after use unless her daughter is obsessively clean. In this case she picks up every spoon and utensil her mother uses, rudely washing it, scrubbing everything within sight and making pointed remarks about hygiene.

Every obscure ingredient imaginable is produced. Recipes are collected. Calories are counted assiduously, scorn being poured upon other people's efforts to lose weight. Infinite care is given to the presentation of food, every dish beautifully decorated and made as tempting as possible for those who are going to eat it – everyone except herself.

Later on, usually in the bingeing and vomiting phase, food begins to disappear from the larder, empty packets and tins are found under beds, in cupboards, under the sofa, behind gramophone records. Mothers are initially relieved, feeling that at least their daughter is eating something. It is tempting, but a great mistake, to deliberately buy food which a daughter might enjoy and leave it around hoping she will eat when she is hungry.

Anorectics are desperately hungry, at least until the illness is well advanced, but are determined to give in to their appetite as seldom as possible, never in front of people. Their conflict with themselves is terrible, reaching and maintaining nightmare proportions. Many girls talk with despair about the two people in their heads, one telling them to eat and the other telling them not to. As the starvation increases and normal physical and psychological resources are diminished so the horror of the anorectic condition intensifies.

Dieting develops into ritual. Vegetables are cut into tiny pieces, carefully arranged and later eaten at a maddeningly slow pace. The mother who is cooking for everyone else at a normal speed is driven to distraction by this. She becomes increasingly impatient, eventually exploding with anger. The anorectic is secretly delighted, either regarding her mother pityingly or yelling back.

By the time the meal is ready the atmosphere is appalling. Efforts at conversation dwindle, tensions increase. The father, egged on by the mother's martyred expression, loses his temper only to be rounded on by the mother with forceful remarks about his general ineptness. The patient throws a fit and her plate, rushing out of the room leaving behind a boiling pot of bitterness, frustration, guilt and anger.

Constant pressure to eat may be self-defeating. Ignoring the eating problem altogether, as so often advised by people with no experience of anorexia nervosa, is dangerous as it can lead to severe complications. When dieting becomes an illness it has affected a girl both physically and mentally to the point where she is not able to reverse it voluntarily.

It cannot be emphasised too strongly that parents who see their daughter losing weight and exercising frenetically and who are aware of the withdrawal and change of personality, who know their daughter's monthly periods have stopped, who find she makes excuses for missing meals and makes a regular visit to the lavatory immediately after those she does eat, who find she is obsessively interested in food and especially in feeding other people, and for whom every meal is a battleground, should seek help immediately.

A mother may at first be angry at the rejection of her food. Later she realises it is unreasonable for a mother to bully or coax any but the very smallest child to eat. She realises that although dieting is common, the iron determination to lose weight coupled with an obsessive interest in food may indicate that her daughter is ill.

Attempts to deal with this without having a proper diagnosis from a doctor may be dangerous, contributing to a chronic if not fatal illness. Unfortunately anorexia nervosa is an illness which reacts to a need in the mother to be involved and caring. This may be the first opportunity she has had for many years to feel a real sense of purpose. The earlier help is sought, the greater chance there is of a cure.

Delay in seeking help may stem from a parent's fear of mental illness. Anorexia nervosa is a neurosis, not madness. The terrible fear of many sufferers and their families that they are going insane is not justified. They are distressed and desperate. Most of this fear could be removed if only the illness was explained to them more clearly.

Neurosis and neurotic are highly emotive words which people fling around without understanding their meaning. They use them to describe someone, often a woman, for whom they have an irrational dislike. No explanation is normally either asked for or offered and the 'neurotic' is written off as hopeless.

Here are two descriptions of neurosis which parents might find enlightening. The first comes from the writings of Professor Eysenck:

Neuroses are self-limiting, in other words sufferers tend to get better without any form of psychiatric or medical treatment. The extent of spontaneous remission is not always realised, but the consensus of a large number of varied studies may be summed up by saying that on the whole some two out of three neurotics, suffering from fairly serious to very serious disorders, improve greatly or recover completely over a period of two years or so when not receiving any psychiatric treatment. This is a high proportion, and must always be born in mind when assessing the effects of any method or therapy. If people get better by themselves, without treatment, then clearly a particular method of treatment must do better than that. It would not be sufficient to point to a recovery rate of two out of three and claim that this proved the efficacy of the treatment. Different types of neurotic disorder recover at different rates. Neurotics have relative insight into their disorder. The neurotic typically knows that his behaviour is irrational, counter productive and against his own best interests. He does it because he cannot help himself. He has insight into his condition in the sense that he knows

49

perfectly well that something is wrong; he simply cannot do anything to help himself.

The second description, by Jung, gives a rather different understanding of the neurotic condition.

Neurosis is an inner cleavage – the state of being at war with oneself. Everything that accentuates this cleavage makes the patient worse, and everything that mitigates it tends to heal the patient. What drives people to war with themselves is the intuition or knowledge that they consist of two persons in opposition to one another. The conflict may be between the sensual and the spiritual man, or between the ego and the shadow. It is what Faust means when he says 'Two souls, alas, dwell in my breast apart.' A neurosis is a dissociation of personality.

Is neurosis, like greatness, something which some are born to, some acquire and some have thrust upon them? In this case, where do patients with anorexia nervosa stand?

The difficulties are compounded in the case of older (secondary) patients, especially those who have already left home. It may be difficult to persuade a daughter to see a doctor and even when she has done so to accept treatment and help. However, most girls are now sufficiently frightened by the implications of the illness to consult a doctor eventually. They are often already run down and debilitated, as the onset of anorexia nervosa can follow an unhappy love affair, broken engagement, change of job, or an abortion. It also frequently accompanies a tremendous effort to take and pass A-levels and university entrance examinations, or to hold down an uncongenial or difficult job, possibly involving leaving home for the first time.

These secondary patients are more likely to binge and vomit than to abstain and starve. When alone they eat enormous quantities of food, spending any money they have on food which they gorge rapidly only to throw up again.

When at home they raid the larder, making orderly house-keeping impossible for the mother. The mother's constant uncertainty of knowing whether she is going to be able to feed her family that night as she had planned rapidly increases the tensions between mother and daughter.

These are also heightened by the anorectic's fear and distress at her lack of control. The vomiting is usually surreptitious, but occasionally bags of vomit are stored in cupboards and under beds for the mother to dispose of. This is not only disgusting but is completely out of character for girls who are hyper-fastidious, obsessively clean and who are apt to regard the entry of a sibling or parent into their bedroom as a gross violation of privacy.

Once the illness has taken hold, a mother finds her daughter wishes to be with her constantly. She never leaves her, asking for her advice on every subject and then rejecting it. This makes the mother feel trapped and helpless. She begins to avoid her daughter at the very time her daughter desperately needs to be given the opportunity to talk out her worries and conflicts.

The anorectic girl is jealous of the time her mother spends with her siblings. Her attempts to annex her mother completely, while at the same time apparently doing everything she can to hurt and upset her, angers and alienates them. Her isolation naturally increases to the point where the only human contact permanently available to her is that with her mother. Even mothers who are aware of the increasing and unhealthy mutual involvement are not able to find any way to stop this process. Some mothers try to cope with it by finding a job, embarking on a degree course or by becoming involved with something, anything, outside their homes.

Every mother with an anorectic daughter is familiar with the moments when, irritated almost beyond endurance, she suddenly turns and unexpectedly sees her daughter standing there – frail, dejected, cold, her face green and gaunt, pleading silently for love and compassion. The mother's

51

heart turns over, her stomach twists, her commitment to the happiness and health of her most vulnerable child is re-affirmed. The detachment and compassionate uninvolved understanding which her daughter so desperately needs from her are one step further off.

3

Causes

It were infinite to judge causes or the causes of causes.

Francis Bacon

The possible causes of anorexia nervosa, include factors which would not upset a basically secure adolescent. The personality and general health, both physical and psychological, of an anorectic must also play a significant part in the onset and development of anorexia nervosa.

REJECTION OF PUBERTY AND A FEAR OF GROWING UP

The rejection of puberty and a fear of growing up are the most commonly given causes of anorexia nervosa. The possible reasons for rejecting puberty include a fear of having to be emotionally and financially independent and self-supporting and of having to face the implications of men, sex and marriage. This last fear may be a reflection of the mother's experiences and attitudes, of possible disappointments, dissatisfactions and resentments.

A woman who is happy in her domestic role is unlikely to sour or alarm her daughter into taking fright and flight. Some anorectics feel overpowered by their mothers, although mothers cannot see why this should be so. The girls are terrified of competing with their mothers and feel hopeless and helpless at the prospect. They see their mothers as 'good' and themselves as 'bad'. If they can avoid growing up, no demands will be made upon them. The strength of their fear means they do not have to make a conscious decision to retreat from maturity, their subconscious takes control, making the decision for them.

Fear and disgust of menstruation and sex are mentioned as important factors, deriving at least in part from their early impressions of their mothers' feelings about them. Many of the mothers suffer from pre-menstrual tension and from cyclical migraine, many of them are approaching the menopause at the same time their daughters are reaching puberty. Mothers may be subconsciously jealous of their daughters' ability to have children and to embark on adult life with the hopes the mothers once had, at the very time they are themselves relinquishing some of their own female functions. The whole area may be fraught with difficulties and tensions.

It seems that mothers forget to tell their daughters about the enormous satisfactions and pleasures a woman can gain from the bearing and rearing of children and a happy marriage. Like mothers without an anorectic daughter, some women have found marriage unrewarding, sexually frustrating, and resent the demands made upon them by their husbands and families.

The daughters' impressions that their mothers gave them no information about sex is not borne out by the mothers' distinct recollections of having done so. Sex instruction which is given in nearly all schools coupled with the often more satisfactory and explicit information gleaned in the school playground and dormitory, make it increasingly unlikely any girl could reach puberty in total ignorance. She may have deliberately avoided listening when sex and menstruation were discussed. Some girls, particularly the shy and inhibited, find bleeding frightening and disgusting and the tummy aches unbearable. It is easier and less embarrassing to discuss all this with their contemporaries than with their mothers. Mothers were prepared to answer questions but their daughters never asked any. This may have been due to the nature of their relationship.

CHANGE OF SCHOOL OR MOVE OF HOUSE

A change of school appears to be a precipitating cause only when it involves moving from a primary school to a secondary school either in a different area or without the company of at least one friend from the previous school. The loss of a best friend with whom anything can be discussed and of acceptance by one another's family can be serious, especially at puberty. It may have been difficult for a girl to reach the academic standard necessary for entry to the school of her parents' choice. She lives in the constant fear of not being able to maintain this. There are anorectics at boarding schools who would be far happier at home. Girls may be sent to boarding school because it is felt that parental difficulties, amounting to an actual or impending divorce, make it better for them to be away from home. The reverse is often the case. Girls away from home can suffer from overwrought imaginings, the uncertainty being more frightening than reality. Girls may feel protective towards their mothers and therefore hurt by their inability to give their mothers comfort and support at a difficult time.

Moving house can represent major stress for any or all members of a family. It may involve changing school and the father changing or losing his job. The mother is busy and worried. She may feel lonely and isolated and not be as aware as usual of her daughter's unhappiness and need for reassurance.

PARENTAL DISCORD

Where would psychiatrists be without it? In all families there are discords, arguments, tensions, but it is the underlying, denied or hidden conflicts which are thought to be so destructive in the family of an anorectic. This is supported by the remarkably low divorce rate in these families – 12 per cent as opposed to the 30 per cent national average. Children who develop anorexia nervosa are highly sensitive and acutely perceptive, and so may be aware of slow-burning dissatisfactions and parental strains other children might miss. They become disheartened, the time between puberty and independence seeming interminable. The prospect of 'waiting in the wings' for several years can seem bleak to a child who can see no hope of any amelioration of the armed truce between her parents. A retreat into ill-health is one way of passing the time.

Divorce is increasingly common. The sophisticated attitude which many adolescents demonstrate towards it masks their despair and panic at the possibility of a future without a stable base. Children who are highly strung can make themselves sick with apprehension and fear over incidents which they may perceive to be more serious than they really are. Their imaginations run riot, fired by the examples all around them of the havoc and unhappiness a divorce can cause. It is hard to assess whether it is worse for children to live with parents who cannot get on together or to be dragged through a divorce which is bound to affect them even when the parents do their best to 'behave well'.

Anorexia nervosa is in many cases seen as a manifestation of chronic distress within the family. The time and resources may not be available to effect a resolution of any problems, so the best hope is that the anorectic can be held steady until she is mature enough to separate emotionally as well as physically from her family and make a stable life for herself. Major parental discord, whether acted out in terms of separation and divorce or not, is unhappily held to confer a poor prognosis.

FAMILY HEAVILY INVOLVED WITH FOOD, PROFESSIONALLY OR OTHERWISE

This raises the question of the symbolism of eating and fasting, of why one family should use food as the centre of its needs and conflicts. There is an amount of psychoanalytical literature available on this subject. A family which sees their involvement with food as a major factor in their daughter's illness might find reading enlightening. A history of family eating eccentricities is associated with prolonged eating disorders. This adds weight to the theories of those who see anorexia nervosa as the manifestation of chronic food allergy.

MOTHER OVER-CONCERNED WITH HER OWN APPEARANCE

This assertion infuriates mothers. A mother feels she is being accused of being obsessed with her appearance to the detriment of her family and of being obsessively concerned with her figure and therefore her weight. If she does not pay attention to her appearance it will be taken as an indication of underlying depression and deemed to be one of the causes of her daughter's illness. Girls who develop anorexia nervosa are sometimes said to come from good-looking families who are supposed to spend undue time and effort achieving this effect. Good looks are an accident of birth, and cleanliness and good grooming merely habits with which the mother can see nothing wrong. What is actually meant is an over-concern with the appearance of the family, sartorially, socially, academically, domestically. The keeping up of appearances, conforming too rigidly to conventional standards are the trouble. The inference is that individuality and self-expression are regarded most unfavourably, found unacceptable and repressed so severely that a daughter who is unable to express herself openly develops anorexia nervosa as a defence.

MATERNAL DEPRESSION

This implies a depression which leads to a mother's withdrawal from and lack of tolerance for the problems of her teenage daughter. It is measured by the presence of at least three of the following; depression of mood, sense of help-lessness and irritability, loss of energy and zest and diminu-tion of libido, present for at least six months before signs of anorexia nervosa appeared. It is particularly acute in mothers of patients in the 11–14 age group. A number of mothers clearly suffer from recurrent bouts of depression but these symptoms are also natural reactions for a mother living with an anorectic daughter. Memory and precise dating of mood are notoriously unreliable. A mother feels under at-tack when categorised as depressed. She feels this implies a lack in her personality which leads her to neglect her chil-dren, and which worse still may be hereditary. A doctor who has no experience of living with and looking after an anorec-tic cannot understand the constant strain and draining of resources and energy involved. Depression, like guilt, can be an easy excuse for the mother, an easy way out for the doctor, and may thereby mask something more serious. The mother is probably worried sick and exhausted, struggling with her own anxiety and the need to keep going at all costs. She could hardly be expected to be euphoric. Unfortunately some mothers find themselves being pressurised into admit-ting constant depression, in order to fit in with a doctor's pet theories.

OTHER FAMILY PROBLEMS: I.E. FATHER'S LOSS OF JOB, ILLNESS OF PARENT OR SIBLING

All these represent extra strain on a mother and result in her decreasing the attention she usually gives to other members of the family. A daughter who is sensitive and caring, as are all anorectics, may shelve or conceal her own unhappiness and distress until she herself needs help and extra attention. She feels too guilty about the additional strain this would impose on her mother to mention it. The prolonged illness, commonly a mental or physical handicap, of a sibling always creates difficulties for other children in a family. A daughter

58

may suffer from intense jealousy, feeling neglected at the extra attention her mother and father give to the ill child. She may be afraid that she could give birth to a handicapped child if she were to marry and have children. This is another reason why she might find the implications of puberty frightening and unacceptable. She is often ashamed of her sibling and suffers from teasing and taunting at school. There may be an element of competition in her development of anorexia nervosa, perfectly understandable in the circumstances, her illness being an attempt to attract more attention and care.

The father's loss of his job inevitably leads to insecurity, financial worries, tensions, parental squabbling. The mother has her husband at home all day, restless and worried. There may be endless disappointments as he is turned down from one job after another. Fathers naturally find it hard to change course in middle age. Sometimes a rapid and radical readjustment involving a totally different and reduced lifestyle will be necessary for the whole family. This may involve the move of school or house which has already been seen as presenting major difficulties for some adolescents.

PARENTAL ILLNESS

The incidence of psychiatric ill-health in the parents of patients with anorexia nervosa is well documented. One survey discloses that 24 per cent of patients had at least one parent who had been treated for psychiatric problems at some time during their marriage, 8 per cent had depression, mainly of a neurotic kind, 8 per cent had anxiety/phobic states, 2 per cent suffered from manic depression, 5 per cent were alcoholics, 1 per cent had a sociopathic disorder. The survey goes on to say that three-quarters of the young patients' mothers were considered to be depressed prior to the onset of anorexia nervosa and nearly half the spouses of these women were also depressed to some degree.

Although it is recognised that the incidence of physical

illness is greater than average in the parents of psychiatrically ill children, the mothers of patients with anorexia nervosa usually describe themselves as physically strong apart from their frequently chequered obstetric history.

Any form of ill-health within a family involves the mother in additional work and worry and the need to devote extra attention to the sick member. Surveys of parental health will naturally vary depending on the level of disturbance and chronicity of patients included in any one study.

DEATH OF PARENT, GRANDPARENT OR SIBLING

The distress caused by the death of a parent is self-evident, whether or not this is complicated by guilt resulting from ambivalent feelings towards the parent when they were alive. The other parent, usually the mother, can become over-dependent on the children of the marriage. She may be unable to express grief properly, preventing the family coming to terms with the loss and making the painful readjustment necessary for a normal life to be resumed. The anorectic, with her tendency to take other people's burdens upon herself, is swamped and finds refuge in illness.

The death of a grandparent is traumatic for potential anorectics. They badly need the security of an extended family, and a grandparent often has time to listen to a grandchild's problems when the parents are too busy. A long illness or family dissension preceding the death may have been harrowing. Mourning may be difficult so that feelings are bottled up with consequent damage to the mourners. It is easy to overlook and underestimate children's grief. Parents who felt a daughter had recovered well from a death because she showed no visible signs of being upset might have missed the point badly.

The early death of a sibling, either after or before the birth of the anorectic, and the stillbirths and miscarriages which appear common in the families are thought by some healers to be the major cause of anorexia nervosa. Girls may feel they were born to compensate and therefore good behaviour and special consideration towards their mothers are incumbent upon them. Parents are horrified when this is pointed out to them.

EXPECTATIONS OF PATIENTS AND PARENTS, LEADING TO FEAR OF FAILURE

There is considerable division of opinion about this. In a study carried out by a leading expert, only 14 per cent of patients working for examinations were found to be subjected to intense pressure from their parents. Many of the pressures come from within the girls themselves. Anorectics are usually perfectionists, highly conscientious and keen to do well. They mention that while the father is usually ambitious for himself as well as for them, the mother wants them to do all the things she has never done, to succeed where she has not even attempted. This is not always true. They see this vision as encompassing not only academic achievement leading to a successful career, but also the social, moral and sexual freedom which mothers are popularly supposed to feel they have missed.

It is indisputable that the environment and upbringing of girls who develop anorexia nervosa are likely to lead to conscious or unintended pressure on them to perform well in every sphere – 'every one a winner'. The fear of failure intensifies as examinations loom menacingly closer and closer. Whatever the attitude and the expectations of parents, a girl's peers and the staff who teach her are naturally competitive and generate a competitive atmosphere. Girls with additional difficulties in their home circumstances are unable to face the trials of the enormous effort and hard work which will be demanded of them if they are to succeed, and so take self-protective refuge in anorexia nervosa.

PREGNANCY OF MOTHER, CLOSE FRIEND OR SIBLING

An adolescent whose mother becomes pregnant finds herself brought face to face with the implications inherent in puberty. Every bodily function is emphasised – impregnation, pregnancy, vomiting, childbirth, pain, breast feeding, babies' nappies. She is forcibly reminded that her mother is, like herself, female, with normal emotional and sexual needs. If her parents' relationship has been inharmonious she may see a striking ambivalence in her mother being physically intimate with a man she does not appear to love deeply. She is also made aware of her father's sexuality. Even in these enlightened days teenagers still find the thought of their parents making love both ludicrous and highly unlikely.

Love and marriage seem unpleasantly complicated, far removed from teenage romantic fantasy of the happiness and fulfilment which they hope for.

Her mother's withdrawal into the lovely haze that comes with a late and longed-for pregnancy arouses resentment. She feels guilty about her reactions, redoubles her efforts to help and look after her mother. By the time the baby arrives the strain of her confusion and natural family anxiety about the health of a baby born to a middle-aged mother have largely drained her own resources at a time when they need to be reinforced. She demands extra mothering, which her mother may be unable to give her until her ill-health ensures it. The family structure which has been disturbed by the new arrival becomes impossible to realign and reorganise satisfactorily.

The mother is torn between the urgent needs of at least two very demanding children and becomes increasingly inadequate. The guilt she feels about her daughter's anorexia nervosa possibly being caused by her arguably self-indulgent and escapist longing for her baby, is made worse by the knowledge that this daughter subconsciously feels the baby should be her own. The family is in disarray. The problems gather momentum. The anorectic also sees her father doting on the baby and feels that she is bereft. The mother can see she has a great deal to do and a great deal to answer for. She will have to find within herself more love and patience than she believes herself to be capable of if this situation is to be resolved and her daughter restored to health.

To a lesser degree, these problems may also arise when a close friend or sibling has a baby. She feels abandoned when the baby arrives and is the centre of attention. The girl who pretended to break her ankle at the christening of her younger sister's baby was acting out her ever-present need to be cosseted and cared for. Most mothers of anorectics come from large families, they are rarely only children, which means they may have too easy an acceptance of difficult inter-family relationships. They may have acquired in their own early childhood the self-protective knack of withdrawing mentally from those around them, of making their own space. They may not always make enough effort to ensure that their children are communicating even if not co-operating with one another, or to make it easier for them to do so.

MOTHER RETURNING TO WORK

This is 'heads I lose, tails you win'. It may be the reasons which impel a woman to return to work which lead to her daughter's anorexia nervosa rather than the actual decision to do so. Psychiatrists who look after patients with anorexia nervosa often make considerable efforts to persuade the mothers to take up work, so they must feel the attendant risks are negligible. They may not believe a woman can be happy and fully occupied looking after her children and husband. It is obviously true that many mothers would benefit from being removed some of the time from the domestic problems which beset them, but added exhaustion and strain will not help them or their daughters. They may need diversion rather than employment.

4

The Search for Help

Honour a physician with the honour due unto him for
the uses which you may have of him: for the Lord hath
created him.

Ecclesiasticus

Once a mother is aware her daughter may have anorexia
nervosa she will set out to find help. This process may be long
and painful. She may be blamed for not having taken her
daughter to the doctor sooner, even though a previous
attempt to do so may have produced no result other than a
suggestion that she is neurotic and over-protective and the
best thing she could do for her daughter is to leave her alone.

The mother of an anorectic is said often to refuse to accept
that her daughter is suffering from anorexia nervosa, although
in the majority of cases it is the mother who notices her
daughter's condition and takes her to the doctor in the first
place. It is undoubtedly true that some parents are deeply
ashamed of having a daughter who is wasting away and
whose eating habits are out of their control. They are frightened by the unfortunate misconceptions and publicity which
surround the illness and its treatment. They deny even the
possibility of having a daughter with anorexia nervosa – that
is something which only happens to other people.

Sometimes the weight loss is noticed during a visit to the
surgery for some other reason, enabling the doctor to bring
up the subject and see if help would be acceptable. Occasionally a talk with a doctor in whom she has confidence can help

to prevent a girl who is on the brink of serious anorexia nervosa from taking it any further. Unfortunately the five-minute appointments in many large group practices, combined with the resulting lack of a satisfactory, or indeed any, relationship between patient and doctor, mean that a girl may not receive the support, understanding and regular medical supervision which might reverse the illness.

Doctors, too, may be unwilling to admit that a patient of theirs could be anorectic. Nor do they always seem able to recognise the illness. 'Allow your mother to prepare some prunes and custard for you, eat it up and you will be well on the way to recovery' betrays the absence of even the vaguest understanding of the condition. Fortunately the increasing interest in anorexia nervosa, is making early diagnosis much more common.

When a mother describes her daughter's state in a way which makes it quite clear to her GP that she is referring to anorexia nervosa it is pointless for him to sit silent, allowing a knowing smile to flit across his face, and then to maintain later that the mother was unwilling to accept his unspoken diagnosis. He must explain to her what the symptoms are and why he thinks her daughter has anorexia nervosa. They can discuss what the next steps might be and decide what to do.

If the mother is certain her daughter has anorexia nervosa there is no reason why she should not herself produce a description of the symptoms for the doctor's benefit. There are books about anorexia nervosa at most public libraries which contain plenty of medical information, including descriptions and names of drugs used to treat the condition with descriptions of their effects and possible side-effects.

The GP may wish to avoid unnecessary drama and alarm, feeling that a mild case will probably clear up if a firm watch is kept upon the patient and that a holding operation is all that is required. The potential anorectic may simply get over the hurdle which seems temporarily insurmountable. Exams may be taken and passed, a new interest or boy friend appear upon the scene and the danger point is passed.

Mothers ask whether a GP can handle the illness without recourse to consultant help. The answer seems to be that he can, provided:

1. He detects the illness fairly early on.
2. He takes a consistently firm line with the patient as far as her eating habits are concerned and is prepared to remove the responsibility of overseeing these from her mother.
3. He has the available time and necessary commitment to spend time every week when he weighs her, talking to her about anything he thinks may be worrying her.
4. He can be responsible for weighing her.
5. He is willing to give her school or college any necessary instructions about her meals and how she should be treated.
6. He has the co-operation and support of her parents.

If a mother knows her daughter will be angry if her thinness is commented on she can always think up some excuse to visit the doctor, having telephoned or written to him in advance. He will be able to contrive to see her daughter alone and talk to her about the possibility of anorexia nervosa without an unseemly fight between mother and daughter breaking out in the surgery. Some doctors feel that the large number of eating problems with which they are presented is becoming out of proportion, firm handling being all that is needed. When these problems do not represent a cry for help they are probably right.

It is not only with anorexia nervosa but with a great many complaints involving her children that the relationship between mother and doctor may represent real and serious difficulty. The basis of the trouble between mothers and doctors seems to be a fundamental inability to accept each other's genuine concern for the health and welfare of the patient.

A certain amount of misunderstanding arises because although their aims are the same, the objectives are rather different. The doctor's job is to restore the girl's health and strength so she may resume normal life as soon as possible. The mother takes a wider view, seeing her daughter's illness in the context of her future. She is naturally anxious that she should recover completely both physically and mentally so that she will be able to lead a full and independent life once she is old enough to do so. This is particularly relevant to anorexia nervosa as it is an illness which can become chronic.

The doctor knows it is perfectly reasonable for a mother to feel like this – he would be the first to condemn her if she did not. The mother knows that if she knew more than the doctors her daughter would not need them in the first place. A mother who is experiencing real difficulty in communicating with her daughter's doctor might find it helpful to discover his attitude to mothers in general and to his own in particular as she will then be able to understand and make allowances for his prejudices.

There sometimes seems to be an element of competition between mothers, doctors and other members of the caring professions. Mothers feel they are automatically blamed for anything wrong with their children but are unable to do anything practical to help as no one will tell them what to do. A mother may be so enraged by a doctor that she is driven to wonder what he has done to his own children that makes him so eager to protect other people's from their parents.

The dissatisfaction people feel with the medical profession is partly due to the unreal and unfulfillable demands made on them by a general public which has been educated to expect miracles which the doctors are unable to perform. The function of doctors is to treat, not necessarily to cure, although this is a consummation devoutly to be wished.

People enter the so-called caring professions for a wide variety of reasons, some of which involve looking after other people. The same can be said of mothers and marriage.

The mother whose daughter has anorexia nervosa feels at a considerable disadvantage because of what she feels appears to be a failure of mothering on her part. The doctor feels under pressure to succeed where she has failed, knowing he may eventually have to refer the patient to a consultant who has wide experience of dealing with anorexia nervosa.

Doctors must try to understand that mothers have been worried and under strain for some time before the condition is diagnosed. Mothers know doctors are overworked, well-intentioned people who are doing their best to help their patients, and that anorexia nervosa is a complex and difficult illness for which no instant cure exists.

There is no doubt that many GPs dislike handing a child who has been a patient for most, if not all, of her life on to a psychiatrist. When this is coupled with a well-intentioned wish to avoid labelling a girl with an illness which has unfortunate connotations, frustration, misunderstanding and delay are almost inevitable.

Psychiatry is the Cinderella of the medical profession, regarded by many doctors, including responsible psychiatrists, as a last hope rather than as a first line of defence. The scepticism of the general public is partly due to the lack of obvious and dramatic success such as results from surgical intervention or medication. Psychiatrists know that at present cure is unlikely, sometimes impossible, for a proportion of their patients. The best they can do for many neurotic and psychotic patients is to ensure that their condition can be contained within limits which make normal life either totally or partially possible.

To the uninitiated the psychiatrist's greatest difficulty lies not in any God-like image he may appear to wish to project but in the superhuman demands he is forced to make upon himself in order to be able to face the needs and demands of his patients. He is his own worst enemy, treading warily through the minefields of other people's emotions with the constant possibility of being finally blown up by his own.

The three criteria quoted for a career in psychiatry are a wish to be of service to others, an overwhelming curiosity about other people and an intense need to be needed. Added to these should be a generous spirit, compassion and constructive understanding.

Any woman who has ever stretched out her nerveless hand for a strong cup of coffee after an hour spent listening to a distraught friend on the telephone knows there is nothing more frustrating and exhausting than listening to other people's apparently insuperable problems. Nothing is more wearying than trying to suggest solutions to these problems when the people concerned do not listen, appearing curiously reluctant to find answers. It is hard for the layman to accept that these difficulties may give a pattern and stability of a sort; without their problems many people would be in a worse state than they are with them. The constant listening is what psychiatrists do most of the time. The draining of their own resources which this entails and the depressing effect it has on some of them is more than most mothers of anorectics would be able or prepared to tolerate.

Psychology and its allied trades are increasingly felt to have largely replaced common sense. Many mothers think they might do better with their children if they could have the confidence to rely less on 'experts' and more on mother wit. There are many parents who have come to feel that a sharp slap on the bottom or ten minutes in the corner had faster and less emotionally damaging consequences than tortuous enquiries as to why a small child might enjoy throwing stones through windows or plucking the budgerigar.

Certainly for many people psychological jargon and mystique are simply a defensive manoeuvre to defend a discipline which has gathered a hold in the same way as any creed which uses guilt as its basis. Mankind survived for a remarkably long time on religion and philosophy before the advent of Freud and his confrères. It is valid to see the rise of psychiatry as a device that enables Western man to maintain at least a minimal equilibrium and some sort of status quo during the difficult period of transition from the ending of the tyranny of the consumer durable to the beginning of the Glass Bead Game.

Many mothers have initially strong reactions to a psychiatrist who is caring for – or apparently interfering with – any member of their family. Some, and these are in the minority, are only too happy to have the burden removed from their own shoulders, meekly accepting the blame, grateful to anyone who is able and willing to mediate between them and their daughters. They show a gratifying faith in a doctor's ability to look after their daughter, accepting what they are told without question. They are enormously relieved at being able to hand over this difficult problem to someone else. Should they show any signs of becoming tiresome and asking awkward questions they can be easily calmed with firm reassurance and the odd compliment ('such a nice man, so understanding, so attractive').

The other more usual type of mother is a different proposition. She will demand a precise definition of her daughter's illness and its likely duration and outcome. Doctors see this as a lack of trust in their professional ability rather than as understandable concern. This mother will be labelled as difficult and aggressive.

Doctors often find mothers of anorectics tiresome to deal with. They do not, as one mother so aptly put it, 'go away singing if the doctor smiles at them'. They are more likely to go away baffled and worried because their questions are evaded or dismissed and all they can see is that their daughter is getting worse. They would feel totally irresponsible if they did not do their best to find out what was going on. They are continually frustrated by being treated as their daughter's arch-enemy when all they are concerned about is her welfare.

This mother needs to have all the information possible because it is only by facing and understanding the situation that she is able to decide on the best way to help her daughter and to stick to it. It is as pointless for the doctors to prevaricate with this mother as it would be for the enraged mother to speculate about the type of doctor who finds absorbing interest and satisfaction in bullying and cajoling attractive adolescent girls.

She may be afraid that the psychological aspects of the treatment will disclose facts about her own life which she might prefer to stay hidden. This may produce an attitude towards her which she feels is hostile and unhelpful to her daughter and yet she knows that to waste the doctor's time with excuses, however justified, will do nothing to help her daughter.

Medical opinion is divided among those who see anorexia nervosa as a manifestation of a conflict which began at or before infancy and others who feel that the root cause is likely to be of more recent origin. Some maintain that the more serious the disorder the earlier must have been the disturbance between mother and child.

The mothers themselves, with the mixed benefits of plenty of experience but no knowledge apart from their gut instinct, nearly all felt at some time that this particular daughter was likely to find adolescence difficult. A surprisingly large number were aware that anorexia nervosa was the most likely path for her to take.

Some mothers suffered from the illness during adolescence and could see the possibility of the pattern repeating itself. Others thought a constant difficulty in feeding this daughter had alerted them to the danger of any adolescent conflict centring on food. A mother is reluctant to mention this to a doctor as she may be told, or given to understand, that she was obviously obsessed with the idea of anorexia nervosa, driving her daughter into it.

Most mothers have far more sense and insight than they are given credit for, although it must be very hard for a doctor to accept this when he is presented with a daughter who has spent all her childhood with her mother and whom he sees to be in a state ranging from obvious emaciation to almost total mental and physical collapse. A doctor can be so obsessed with his own theories he overlooks factors which he ought to register.

Doctors are so used to blaming the mother for her sins and omissions that they sometimes forget they are also open to criticism. The mother who after a long-awaited hour-long talk with a consultant psychiatrist heard her very emaciated daughter being told to, 'Go home at once, dear, and find out the difference between an amoeba and a virus. Get your mind on that and you will feel much better', was not unique. She had to make further efforts to contact another doctor, much to the annoyance of her GP, knowing that any mother who changes her daughter's consultant so quickly is automatically seen as difficult and neurotic.

Incidents like this are awkward and mothers are not at all clear about their rights. The National Consumer Council produces an excellent book called *Patients' Rights*, which sets out clearly the rights and responsibilities of patients and doctors in the NHS. It can be obtained from Community Health Councils. MIND, National Association for Mental Health, 22 Harley Street, London W1N 2ED, produce a patients' rights handbook, giving advice and information about the law relating to psychiatric patients.

Mothers are afraid that even the most experienced psychiatrist may not be able to see all sides of the problem, particularly at the initial interview, and may make assumptions based on established theories, which may be dangerous and incorrect. They are concerned that the concentration on the psychological aspects of anorexia nervosa may mean that important medical facts are overlooked. This is not as far-fetched as it sounds. When an anorectic patient in a psychiatric hospital contracted measles a GP had to be called in as none of the doctors in the hospital was able to recognise the illness.

Parents feel they have no real opportunity to explain or discuss their own point of view and their daughter's previous

72

history. They feel condemned without trial on circumstantial evidence. This is not good enough. If it resulted in the condition being reversed and the patient being cured they would be more able to bear it. Occasionally parents see the attack on themselves as a measure of the doctor's inadequacy in dealing with anorexia nervosa. They feel that if a drug were found which could control and cure the illness, no more would be heard of the parents' and especially the mothers' role in anorexia nervosa.

Not all psychiatrists are mischief-making megalomaniacs, just as not all mothers of anorectics are neurotic to the point of being 'nuts'. The mother of a child with a psychosomatic illness is always vulnerable to hostile criticism. A psychiatrist invariably stresses the environmental factor against the genetic one. Equally, psychiatry is also hedged about with distrust, those who practise it tending to be regarded with suspicion by those who do not. 'Extraordinary sort of chap to be a trick-cyclist. Seems perfectly normal' – a father's description of a well-known psychiatrist which neatly sums up current attitudes. It is difficult to assess to what extent psychiatry, like homoeopathy, depends for its therapeutic effect on 'sympathetic magic' – the treating of like with like.

The general distrust is heightened by the heady aura of eroticism surrounding psychiatry and psychoanalysis. Englishmen, less involved with their minds and their mistresses than most other Western races, are deeply suspicious of its effects. The whole thing has far too much to do with sex in their view. What could be more unhealthy than a woman lying horizontal on a couch revealing to a man whose own motives they feel to be at the best dubious and at the worst a mirror image of their own were they in a similarly promising position, secrets and emotions which she has felt unable to express in the marriage bed or to disclose to her mother, lover or best friend. The unfair picture that all too easily emerges is of unscrupulous men taking financial advantage of a series of silly women.

73

There is no doubt that many girls and women find the instant intimacy stimulating. Their emotions are aroused by being able to talk to a member of the opposite sex on a deeper level of understanding and acceptance than they may have previously encountered. This is in itself a telling commentary on Anglo-Saxon attitudes towards women.

He is dominant and detached, she is submissive and subjective, he is professional and she is personal. It was Shakespeare who provided the words which so succinctly describe the undemanding allure of the psychiatrist's couch:

> Hereafter, in a better world than this,
> I shall desire more love and knowledge of you.

As You Like It, Act I, Scene II

Many people would not be able to survive without the help and understanding of their psychiatrist, others need drugs to remain stable. There are also those who find the world in which we live so demanding and stressful they decide the only way to continue is by making a journey into themselves. Unfortunately psychiatry contains an element of 'bought friendship' which renders it open to criticism.

Psychiatrists, unlike other doctors, have occasionally to reveal something of themselves, their interests, personalities and inclinations, in order to establish the mutual trust which enables their patients to do the same. This can lead to dangerous misunderstanding but much of the mistrust surrounding psychiatry stems from the concept of transference.

Is transference a morally sound, therapeutically justified manoeuvre or is it the ultimate dirty trick? Is it the attempt of a frail ego to impose upon a frailer one an unbreakable domination, often with continuing financial reward and a satisfying boost to the morale of the practitioner? Or is it the unavoidable result, especially with anorectics, of tendering the support of a parental figure, with all that implies but

74

without the taboo on incest? The answer depends on the personality and ethics of the doctor concerned.

A mother can hardly fail to present badly when she eventually meets the psychiatrist to whom her daughter has been referred, as by that time her daughter's illness will be worsening and may even be critical. She may find it difficult to face the suggestions being thrown at her about her daughter's illness and her own part in it. Her prolonged worry and the physical and mental exhaustion which it engenders may make her liable to over-react to questions which sound more hostile than is intended.

She is usually told that a difficult family situation is a common contributory factor in anorexia nervosa. If she has in fact been trying to deal with a failing and unhappy marriage she may be made to feel this is the worst thing she could have done. She may also be told it is essential to continue with this unhappy state of affairs as any additional upheaval could have a disastrous effect on her daughter.

The mother may have to make a long journey with a recalcitrant and ill daughter and then have to wait for some time before being seen. Hospital appointment systems are notoriously erratic. It is not unusual for a mother to arrive for an appointment to be told it has had to be cancelled or altered. The performance then has to be repeated. It is sensible to telephone the hospital the day before the visit to make sure there is no misunderstanding about the arrangements.

She should take with her some notes on her daughter's medical history and anything else she considers relevant, in case the notes from her GP or previous hospital have been lost or mislaid. Doing this will also help her to clear her mind and save everyone time and irritation.

At the initial interview a nervous and confused mother may appear defensive and aggressive. She hopes for more reassurance than it is possible to give her. The course of anorexia nervosa is seldom smooth. It may require several hospital admissions, years of care, wear and tear. It affects all members of a family in different ways, all of which compound the problem.

The mother is unlikely to take in everything she is told. She is searching her mind for all the questions she meant to ask, while the hard-pressed doctor is patiently trying to tell her what he thinks she needs to know. She feels blamed for her daughter's anorexia nervosa. This is an illness in which criticism is inherent in the condition.

She must be frank with the doctor since the impressions of the family interaction which he gains at the diagnostic interview may determine his approach to the patient. Nothing is to be gained by concealing family difficulties, marital or financial problems or anything which might affect the anorexia nervosa.

No matter how brilliant and respected her daughter's doctor may be and no matter how reassuring his reputation, he can do very little if the mother is unwilling to face and discuss realistically what he may perceive to be some of the contributing factors. It will be more difficult for him to help her daughter without her co-operation.

There are reasons other than neurotic defence why a mother might fail to reveal details of her private life or that of other members of her family. She may forget small happenings which were not as important to her as they seem in retrospect to have been to her daughter. She may not feel able to trust a stranger when time is too limited to establish any sort of confidence. She may feel his attitude is unfairly critical and likely to damage her relationship with her daughter.

She may think, with justification in the case of a psychosomatic illness, that the information she painfully gives him will not be confidential, as he will think it necessary for the teams of doctors, nurses and social workers with whom he works to know as much about the patient as he does. She may feel her daughter will glean from the questions information which will hurt her. Anorectics are both perceptive and hypersensitive and easily pick up trains of thought.

There are two more reasons why she may conceal information, either deliberately or inadvertently. The first of these is loyalty – a concept apparently unknown to many psychiatrists. The other is retribution – she has to live with the husband and children whom she may have described in less than glowing terms.

Everyone is vulnerable to something or someone at some time during their life. In a mutually dependent family with its complicated interactions, it is normal and right to defend and protect each other's weaknesses against outsiders, except when one or more members of the family is being damaged by doing so.

Occasionally a consultant is driven by what he perceives in a mother–daughter relationship to subject the mother to a devastating personal attack, based more on intuition than information. She cannot answer easily, or even at all, and the unfortunate consequence is likely to be the removal of her daughter from the doctor's care. A process is set in motion whereby the anorectic is moved from doctor to doctor by her increasingly sensitive and desperate mother, with little if any amelioration of her illness.

When mother and daughter first meet the psychiatrist to whom she has been referred he may recommend her daughter be admitted to hospital immediately, depending on the severity of her condition and the availability of beds. More often he suggests her daughter should go home for a week to see if she can begin to put on weight by herself. This is seldom effective, but gives time for the patient and family to adjust to the possibility of a fairly lengthy stay in hospital. Doctors prefer the anorectic girl to say that she *wants* to get better and is willing to come into hospital.

Occasionally a girl is so horrified or so helped by the initial interview that she goes home and starts eating immediately. This is most likely in the minor cases or in the initial stages.

At the first interview the mother should ask exactly what the treatment will entail, whether her daughter will be given any drugs, and what the so-called 'reward' system involves. The family can then discuss realistically what lies ahead.

Parents would sometimes feel happier and less to blame if treatment could be carried out on an out-patient basis. Until recently it was felt admission to hospital was essential in all but the mildest cases. However, the increasing incidence of anorexia nervosa unmatched by an increase in beds or specialised units is leading to a reversal of this view.

Some psychiatric hospitals now feel that out-patient treatment can be as good as in-patient, even in severe cases, depending on the age of the sufferer and the length of time she has had the condition. Others feel that it will only work if the family as a whole is seen twice a week and the patient is seen daily.

Regular family therapy may be considered necessary if out-patient treatment is to be effective, focusing initially on strengthening the marital relationship rather than on the anorexia nervosa. This is important for acute primary (11–15) patients, who need strongly united parents against whom to fight. They need someone outside the family who is available to give them support and guidance when they are overwhelmed and terrified. This is where the psychiatrist or therapist has an important function. In this way weight may be slowly gained. A reasonable weight must be established before psychiatric help can be effective.

'Make sure you keep the upper hand over your parents', is a remark guaranteed to arouse parents' hostility. It is never explained to parents that their daughter needs to be encouraged to start a fight with them which it is essential she should lose. It is only by doing so that she can be quite sure they are stronger than she is and that she is therefore 'safe' with them.

It is not until she is convinced they are in control both of all their children and the family feeding that she is able to slowly relinquish the control she has established over herself and everyone else. Feeding is a parental responsibility and must be in the hands of parents so their children are free to fill their own roles.

78

The initial interview is nearly always tense and may be harrowing. Parents may deny both the anorexia nervosa and the existence of family difficulties. The doctor may need to heighten the parental anxiety to the point of anguish to make them understand how seriously ill their daughter is. Fathers have a greater difficulty than the mother in accepting this. This technique may make a father so angry he will at last take upon himself some of the responsibility for controlling his daughter's eating.

Doing this makes it easier for him to give his wife open support rather than constant criticism. He may at last understand that she is fighting for her daughter's life against her daughter's will and is not simply an uncontrolled sadist. It proves to his daughter that he is genuinely concerned about her and unafraid of her dislike.

To the mothers, doctors can seem to have an elevated view of their own supportive role, unaware that they find the psychiatric kiss and kick technique alarming and bewildering. Common politeness may prevent a mother telling a doctor what she thinks about anorexia nervosa, either subjectively or objectively. She may find her direct questions are evaded. It is easier and probably more helpful to take an intelligent interest in what a doctor is saying, appearing to accept that he is right. During their occasional meetings the doctor is likely to run the conversation on general lines, knowing any of his comments which come uncomfortably close to the mark will be met with blank amazement or outraged denial. The mother has a vague feeling of being persecuted, but feels he is doing his best to help although unfortunately unable to be constructively specific.

At the end of the statutory half-hour the doctor is bristling and baffled. Surely this wretched woman is capable of grasping at least the general direction of his remarks? She is exasperated. Surely this half-witted man is capable of giving her what she is quite reasonably asking for – a straight answer to a straight question. They join in battle instead of uniting in co-operation. His long practice of reaching the door handle first ensures they part politely. She is forced to thank him for his courtesy if not for the consultation, baring her teeth in an agonised smile while restraining an overwhelming desire to push his in.

The dilemma is clear. He cannot tell her what she most needs to know. If he were to do so he would risk breaking the fragile bonds of trust and faith which are his only real weapons in his attempt to cure her daughter. The daughter must feel able to confide in him and to discuss with him problems which worry her and which she feels unable to discuss with her own family, especially her mother. If only mothers could accept that no woman can supply all her daughter's needs, and that if that were possible the daughter would be reduced to being her mother's shadow.

ALTERNATIVE MEDICINE

The present lessening of confidence in conventional medicine leads people with every type of illness to consider the possible advantages of alternative medicine. None of the alternative therapies claims to be able to cure anorexia nervosa, although on the Continent parents have found homoeopathy effective and helpful. These families have always used homoeopathy and so have more trust in it than in other methods. It does not use drugs which may become addictive or have damaging side-effects. Nor is there so much risk of a girl being used as a guinea pig as there is in hospital.

Parents who are dissatisfied with and worried about the methods used to treat their daughter might find it helpful to read *The Alternative Health Guide* by Brian Inglis and Ruth West which gives a description of each type of therapy and addresses of their organisations. Parents who find a particular therapy sympathetic may find it can help their daughter.

Parents might like to contact a practitioner of the therapy

or therapies which they think could help their daughter and discuss the anorexia nervosa with him. An avoidance of any psychological problems of younger girls might be all to the good. The greatest help to a girl might be that in regularly attending a therapist of whatever type she would be able to establish with someone outside her family a rapport which would be supportive and therapeutic. The danger would be that many non-medically trained therapists do not understand the vital importance of weight restoration.

FAMILY THERAPY

There is an increasing trend for every illness with a psychological factor to be regarded as a 'family illness'. The whole lot are sick literally as well as undoubtedly being sick and tired of it. Salvatore Minuchin claims that 'there is no treatment other than family treatment'.

The ecstatic view of some therapists is not matched by that of many parents. A very few families appear to obtain real benefit from family therapy sessions, either in groups of families or singly. They appear to be in the minority.

There are no satisfactory follow-up studies to reassure the wary. Nor are families convinced that there is much point in digging into a family and causing distress if the illness has to run a natural course. The uprooting of 'hidden tensions' may cause things to be said which can never be unsaid and which do not necessarily affect the anorexia nervosa for the better. Husbands and wives feel that rifts are widened, hurts aired, tempers lost, damage done which cannot be undone. A mother may be very distressed by seeing her husband humiliated in front of her.

Parents are most concerned about the effect that therapy sessions have on the siblings. There is a real risk that they may feel blamed for their sister's condition. Other older sisters may take the view that all adolescents are difficult, so

81

what can you expect. Younger ones may do their best to ignore it – probably the best answer for them.

There is concern that once the family therapy has started, the family should have enough sessions. The greatest damage seems to be done when a family is subjected to a few sessions during which a varying amount of unhappiness and distress is stirred up and they are then left high and dry to sort out the resulting muddle themselves.

Parents have grave doubts about any one therapist or team of therapists who seriously imagine that they can alter the interactions in families significantly in this way. Again, the parents and therapists are acting from a different premise and with a different perspective and timescale. If so much can be done to so many by so few in such a short time why are five years of analysis considered necessary for one person?

Parents may also have doubts about the efficacy of a profession which spends so much time monitoring itself. Quite apart from the ridiculous expense of installing television cameras, two-way mirrors, tape recorders – money which might be far better spent in other ways – there is concern that once a structure exists it cannot be dismantled. The technical safeguards – against what? – make confidence unlikely. Even the most feather-brained mother does not have to ask another woman to gawp through her kitchen window to make sure she is scrambling her eggs correctly.

Anorectics vary in their views of family therapy but many of them and their parents feel that a sufferer needs most of all to be treated as an individual. They feel that the concentration on the whole family is wrong for this reason. They feel that the more families are interfered with, analysed and subjected to help, the more uncertain and unstable they become, and the less likely is it that the anorectic can detach herself from them.

Parents are not always clear about their own involvement in a treatment programme. It may mean for all members of the anorectic's family, including much younger siblings, a possibly painful encounter with the anorectic in front of a third party. This will be either singly with the patient or with the whole family together.

The mother does not have to sit with a brave, if tightening, smile, absorbing insults either from her daughter, other members of the family or the doctor or social worker conducting the session. She must say exactly what she thinks and not be afraid to engage in battle with anyone else in the room. She has an important point of view and can do most to help by being frank. Equally, there is no reason for her to escape into a state of shock when she is answered in kind. The time for restraint, consideration and pretending that all is well has long since passed.

In any family with an anorectic member, communication within the family will become increasingly difficult. It may be more marked between siblings, or between the parents with each other or with one or more of their children. The barriers may need to be broken down so that a family can begin to talk and, even more important, to listen to one another. It is lack of time rather than brutality which may make the techniques employed hurtful. Staff may be inexperienced. They are most likely to blunder if the family are putting up a wall of non-cooperation and denial.

The Minuchin definitions of the four types of family which may contain an anorectic member are widely used. Parents might find it helpful to read these. They can identify with other members of their family the category or categories into which their family seems to fall, using this as a basis for discussion. At the beginning of the anorexia nervosa, families may find it hard to tolerate the implied criticisms or to discuss them rationally. It can be helpful for the family to write down their views of these definitions and then to read what one another has written.

According to Salvatore Minuchin the development of psychosomatic illness in a child is related to three factors. They are a special type of family organisation and functioning, involvement of the child in parental conflict, and physiological vulnerability. He feels that the presence of physiological vulnerability in anorexia nervosa is debatable, although others see it as fundamental.

The kind of family functioning involved is characterised by enmeshment, over-protectiveness, rigidity, and a lack of conflict resolution.

Enmeshment – the family members are over-involved with one another and over-responsive, interpersonal boundaries are diffuse, with the family members intruding on each other's thoughts, feelings, and communication. Subsystem boundaries are also diffuse, which results in a confusion of roles. The individual's autonomy is severely restricted by the family system. Anorexia nervosa may hold a family together to prevent individuation and adolescent separation.

Over-protective family – members have a high degree of concern for each other's welfare. Protective responses are constantly elicited and supplied. When there is a sick child, for example, the entire family become involved. Often conflicts are submerged in the process. The child in turn feels responsible for protecting the family.

Rigidly organised families – often presenting themselves as not needing or wanting any change in the family. Preferred transactional patterns are inflexibly maintained.

Lack of conflict resolution – meaning that the family has a low threshold for conflict. Some families simply deny the existence of any conflict. In others, one spouse is a confronter but the other is an avoider. Others bicker but manage to avoid a real confrontation. Issues are therefore not negotiated and resolved. The psychosomatically ill child plays a vital part in the family's avoidance of conflict by presenting a focus for concern. The system reinforces his symptomatic behaviour in order to preserve its pattern of conflict avoidance.

INDIVIDUAL PSYCHOTHERAPY

Psychotherapy varies. A young girl may find relief in talking to someone outside her family about problems and difficulties which are preventing her normal development. An older girl, particularly one with sexual problems who is or has been married, may benefit from the chance to explore these in greater depth. The NHS is unlikely to provide the regular therapy lasting for several years which a trained psycho-therapist would advocate. Unless they have a medical training therapists may be unable to understand or accept why the weight loss needs to be reversed before other therapy is likely to be effective.

There are disadvantages in a girl starting on a course of psychotherapy. It means she is still financially dependent on her parents. It is unlikely she will be able to pay the fees herself if she is still at school or college or starting work. There is no guarantee that in transferring control by her parents to control by a therapist a patient will necessarily achieve the ability to control herself which is fundamental to recovery. There may be less painful, time-consuming and expensive methods of achieving this.

Embarking on a course of psychotherapy inevitably in-creases an anorectic's self-absorption, when what she needs most is to think less about herself, becoming more involved with her contemporaries. It will affect her mobility – she needs to be able to make a break from her immediate environment should an opportunity present itself. It is also likely to reinforce her as being special.

Some anorectics have endured major weight loss during psychotherapy, in some cases life-threatening, and both parents and husbands of anorectics feel bitter about the damage to or death of a daughter or wife.

On the other hand, there is no doubt some girls find greater stability and confidence by having regular contact with someone trained to understand their difficulties. This should, however, be their own decision and at their own expense.

MOURNING AND PRAYER

Healers sometimes feel that the spiritual vacuum in anorexia nervosa stems from the lack of proper mourning in a family. This mourning concerns the death of a member of the family who may or may not be known to the anorectic, or it may point to an unfinished mourning process within the parents, especially the mother, over the death or miscarriage of an earlier child. Dr Kenneth McAll's book *Healing the Family Tree* has been found helpful by parents who see this as a possible cause for their daughter's anorexia nervosa.

'She behaves as though she were possessed by a devil.' The question of possession is inclined to hover over a neurotic illness which defies rational explanation. It is thought that a bond may exist between mother and daughter which leads to the daughter becoming increasingly dependent on her mother and so unable to accomplish the gradual separation necessary for individuation, the daughter therefore being unable to establish her own identity. Healers and psychiatrists differ in one essential about the 'possession syndrome' in that healers recognise that the controlling bond may well have skipped one or more generations whereas psychiatrists are generally unable to envisage a bond other than one between two living people.

Both are agreed that some patients cannot be cured and permanently healed until the bond is broken. Healers see the bondage as being to an ancestor whose death was unmourned or whose funeral was not properly carried out; or to anyone who in the past had a peculiarly malign influence over any member of the family, to anyone whose symptoms are being reproduced in the current sufferer from anorexia nervosa, or, more usually, to an aborted, stillborn, or miscarried baby.

A healer can hold a religious service laying to rest the unquiet spirit inhabiting a girl. It may be that a service which can lay to rest previous children of a mother is most likely to aid the sufferer in that it can cure a long-standing malaise of her mother. Once this has been done, the mother finds that in being released herself the emotional burdens which her anorectic daughter has unconsciously absorbed may be automatically removed.

The suggestion that a healing service might be helpful may be viewed by parents with suspicion and fear. They may have heard of other parents who have attended a service of healing and have been disappointed because there was no obvious 'miracle' cure. Healing has to be done *with*, and not *to*, anyone who needs help. It involves a conscious act of participation on the part of the supplicant coupled with the willingness to accept the need for change within oneself.

Parents sometimes find themselves under well-meant pressure from family or friends to accept that anorexia nervosa is a genuine death wish – the longing for death being part of the inner core of personality which is beyond the help or control of either the sufferer or anyone else. Detachment and understanding on this scale would demand a depth of faith so great that parents would have to accept, even for their own child, death as a new beginning rather than see it as an ending. Most healers do, however, feel that a combination of prayer and hope is undoubtedly effective. The prayer lifts and lightens the burden of guilt from the whole family. The hope may take the form of bribery which provides an incentive for the weight to be restored so that a sufferer is once more able to think rationally and see hope for the future.

Mothers talk of the way their own strong faith has carried them through the worst moments and of the way in which their own prayers and those of others have helped them. A daughter does not always feel able to share her mother's trust in God, rejecting that sure source of help as she does all others. On the other hand, mothers have found great support from their Church, from prayer groups, from the priest, vicar or rabbi. Prayer, like meditation, can provide a break from the turmoil in which a mother can find herself. It enables her to withdraw temporarily and return to the battle refreshed in spirit, mind·and body.

Positive thinking and prayer have a great deal to do with an anorectic's recovery. There are books in every public library which provide useful suggestions for turning negative, harmful thought into positive constructive action.

5

Hospitals

I think it frets the saints in heaven to see
How many desolate creatures on the earth
Have learnt the simple dues of fellowship
And social comfort, in a hospital.

Elizabeth Barrett Browning, 'Aurora Leigh'

This is the first encounter many parents will have had with mental illness. Their first and sometimes continuing reaction to their daughter's anorexia nervosa is a rejection of the psychiatric basis of the disorder. Although an enormous amount of work is being done by mental health organisations to remove the stigma of mental illness there is no doubt that many people still regard it with fear and horror.

This attitude may be dismissed as being based on, 'There, but for the grace of God, go I.' The statement that 'parents and others who find themselves reacting negatively to the very thought that their anorectic relation should see a psychiatrist or enter a psychiatric hospital would perhaps do well to examine their own motives' is intended to annihilate fears that may be based on reasonable doubts.

Unfortunately many mental hospitals are large, frightening Victorian buildings, gloomy inside as well as out. Staff who work there every day may have no idea of the unfortunate effect that the appearance can have on distraught and exhausted parents. Parents are also upset by the sight of the other patients, some of whom are in various states of disturbance.

They feel it may be wrong for a sensitive and sick girl to be with schizophrenics, the old and possibly deranged and incontinent, habitual drug offenders, or those who are hallucinating or seriously withdrawn. They are not receptive to bracing remarks about the need for every member of the community to accept other people as human beings needing help as much as their daughter.

Voluntary workers in psychiatric hospitals talk with concern about the way in which young people with fairly minor problems are admitted and are still there years later, apparently slowly deteriorating. There is no escaping the impression that to some extent these hospitals are regarded as dumping grounds for the socially undesirable.

Against this, the standard of care is usually adequate. There are many people who would not be able to carry on anything even approaching a normal life without psychiatric help of one kind or another, including drugs. The millions of people who swallow sleeping pills, anti-depressants and sedatives every day would be shocked and angry at the idea that they are mentally unwell. Like anorectics they are fundamentally unhappy and unable to come to terms with their life. People who have anorexia nervosa are in the same position but have developed a particularly dangerous and difficult way of coping with their problems.

Admission may cause distress. Girls may be nervous about going into hospital, frightened and rebellious. Mothers are upset when their daughter is taken away from them crying or screaming. They would like to be able to see her tucked up in bed. It is often impossible for the mother to find anyone who can tell her about visiting arrangements or from whom she can discover the best time to telephone the ward to see how her daughter is. Mothers feel that the attitude of the medical staff towards parents of anorectics is hostile. In many cases this is true.

When a mother leaves her daughter at the hospital she experiences a number of conflicting emotions. The first is overwhelming relief coupled with or succeeded by a sickening feeling of bereavement. She thinks that the hospital feels her daughter needs protecting from her. She knows her daughter is going to have to undergo physical and mental changes, some of which will be painful and difficult for her. She knows that she will be criticised behind her back without a chance to explain. A wall of angry resistance and guilt may build up inside her so that even the mildest remark from any of the hospital staff can provoke an outburst of fury. She is for a time overwrought and apprehensive, and usually receives very distressing letters and telephone calls for the first week or so.

With hindsight many girls say that the experience widened their understanding and ability to manage their lives both inside and outside the hospital. The worst problem they had to face was the initial weight gain.

It is therefore of the utmost importance that parents should be clear about the treatment, as once it is under way it is essential they do not interfere or try to alter it. They must be prepared to give the hospital their support, often in the face of their daughter's heart-rending complaints, for a reasonable length of time. If they feel that the treatment plan which has been outlined to them is either inhumane or totally unacceptable then it is imperative they find some other form of treatment. No family and no patient should allow themselves to accept treatment which they know they are likely to reject before it has been given a chance to be effective.

Anorexia nervosa is a long-lasting and unpleasant illness and so are some of the methods of treatment currently available. These are variations of what is known as 'behavioural modification'.

Behavioural modification is the technical name for the well-known bribe and threat technique to which nearly every mother resorts from time to time particularly with small children.

'Stop yelling and you can have an ice cream' is the juvenile version of 'put on 4 kilos and you can have a bath'. Any child psychologist would be only too happy to tell a defaulting mother that this illustrates the desperation, lack of time and ineptitude of the person in control. The only difference between an anorectic and a toddler lies in the fact that an anorectic undeniably has to reach a certain weight before she is able to see the benefits of being well whereas the ice cream provides more immediate pleasure.

This is why the behavioural modification approach is fundamentally weak, open to abuse, and why an intelligent adolescent may not be susceptible to it. This is also why its beneficial effect may not last once the patient has been discharged from hospital, particularly if it has been reinforced with hectoring and bullying of both the patient and her family.

Parents' apprehension may be justified. Hilde Bruch's much quoted remark that the general treatment of anorexia nervosa is so bad that even if the illness itself disappears the psychological after-effects of the treatment are ineradicable, has an element of truth. Many anorectics are certain this is true. Increasing knowledge and understanding of the illness are bringing about an improvement in the medical care. Methods of treatment are less brutal and tube feeding and heavy drugging have largely been abandoned.

The staff and time are not always available to give anorectics the specialised counselling from which they are most likely to benefit and so there is often no alternative to what appear to be shock tactics. There are some hair-raising and authenticated tales of cruelty to anorectics and there is certainly no other illness which arouses such resentment and hostility from both medical staff and the general public.

There can be no defence for some of the experiences which anorectics have had to undergo. These are worse in practice than they sound in print or when described by a doctor to a patient and her mother, couched in vague terms and in a manner which discourages questions. They are unlikely to absorb everything that is said to them, often being prepared to grasp at any straw in desperation.

Even allowing for exaggeration and the aberrations of memory, there is no doubt whatever that some anorectics are subjected to methods which would arouse howls of well-informed protest were they to be applied to political dissidents in the Eastern bloc. There is no adequate excuse for keeping anyone in isolation, lying on a mattress on the floor with nothing to do all day long and nothing to read until an initial weight gain has been achieved. A girl may then be allowed to see a page of a newspaper for a short time and perhaps have a blanket. An anorectic may indeed begin to eat in order to escape from this non-existence. How is she ever going to be able to have anything other than a very jaundiced view of her family for allowing the treatment, a fear and distrust of authority, and an abysmally and permanently low self-esteem for having deserved it?

The medical profession is usually slightly on the defensive but this type of behaviour represents panic. This is understandable when one realises that they are faced with growing numbers of girls suffering from this intractable condition, without any increase in resources and facilities with which to either treat it or carry out large-scale research.

Doctors may be fairly intolerant towards anorexia nervosa, thinking that the anorectics are so defensive, bewildered, hostile and subjective that they are not able to appreciate fully that without this treatment they might be dead. Complaints about the methods employed by individual hospitals seem to such doctors to be self-indulgent.

Another form of treatment offered to anorectics in some special units relies entirely upon refeeding a patient while she is drugged so heavily that she is unable to resist. No psychological help of any kind is attempted. It appears that this is successful, although it may require two or three readmissions, in about half the cases. The other half have an abnormally high mortality rate. It is kill or cure.

The punitive attitude which is sometimes adopted with anorexia nervosa manifests itself in the 'jolt them out of it' school of thought. Anorectics may be put in a terminal cancer ward as it is felt that the sight of 'real' suffering may make them realise how lucky they are not to be in similar straits. They already realise, and the result is a further decline in their minimal self-esteem.

The question is raised, particularly by the anorectics themselves, whether they should be treated in special anorectic units, in a mixed psychiatric ward or in a general medical ward.

Treatment in a general hospital is neither easy to organise nor successful, the only possible exceptions to this being with very young patients in a children's ward. Even here, sisters have been heard to remark that they are here to look after 'sick children'. The implications of naughtiness and non-cooperation do not help but staff are irritated by a child's continuing and apparently unreasonable refusal to eat.

In a ward in a general hospital there are nearly always difficulties. There are too few staff to give undivided attention to patients who seem to be suffering from a self-inflicted illness. If a nurse sits with an anorectic while she eats, it arouses resentment in the other patients. These concern both the inordinate time given to the anorectic and the extra amount of food which some would like to have for themselves. Nursing staff who have not been trained to nurse anorectics are often impatient and angry when a patient will not eat, resenting having to give her proportionately more time and care than they are able to give other patients. After several weeks patients may be thought to be beyond hope and are sent home.

When anorectic girls are in a special anorectic unit there is a tendency for them to try to outdo one another with their descriptions of their symptoms, emotions and unlikely behaviour. They discuss with relish the various ways in which it is possible to outwit the hospital and their parents. They are strikingly resourceful and competitive where methods of losing or controlling their weight are concerned. Both anorectics and their families see that the element of chance in whom they meet in hospital may make a substantial difference to the outcome of the anorexia nervosa once they leave. There is no doubt that information and hints gleaned from other patients contribute to the deterioration of the illness once the anorectic leaves hospital, and to it lasting longer than it would otherwise have done.

In spite of the possible disadvantages, psychiatrists feel that in-patient care is necessary for many anorectics, especially for the young patients whose physical and mental development have been brought to a halt at a critical stage. It is vital for the weight to be restored so that a girl may continue her development. They may be anxious also to remove the patient as soon as possible from the family environment and the endless opportunities for 'games playing' between doctor, patient and family.

However, once a girl is 16 she has the right to choose her own doctor and to refuse to visit a doctor or hospital to whom she has previously been referred. This may mean an anorectic has to be admitted to hospital under Section 3 of the Mental Health Act of 1983 as a life-saving manoeuvre. In many cases the doctor or social worker involved is prepared to sign the order if the parents find the prospect of committing their daughter too painful to contemplate.

Some hospitals now feel it is essential that parents should do this themselves rather than abrogate responsibility to a third party whose ability to help the patient may thereby be considerably reduced. It is important for parents to take this task upon themselves both for their own self-respect and because it is good for the siblings to see that their parents are not afraid to take unpleasant and upsetting action if the welfare of their children demands it.

Once a patient is in hospital, doctors like to enter into a contract with her, always with the reassurance that they will make sure she does not gain too much weight too fast. This is a real and overpowering fear for anorectics. Gaining weight has terrifying implications of losing control over food and attaining mountainous proportions.

If a patient consistently refuses to stick to the contract, even after several readmissions, the problem will be judged to be beyond the capacity of the medical profession and will be handed back to the family to deal with. This is why in anorexia nervosa, more than in any other illness, the family and particularly the mother have to be prepared to play their part in helping the patient to recover, just as they may have to come to accept some degree of responsibility for its development.

Once in hospital, girls are relieved to have the burden of controlling their feeding removed from them, although there may be an initial resistance to altering patterns of behaviour which have evolved over a long time. They feel safe knowing that their welfare is in the hands of experienced staff who understand their behaviour without being shocked or angered by it. Patients with anorexia nervosa need to feel secure in their relationships with other people.

The bed-rest which is sometimes seen by both patients and parents as an iniquitous denial of freedom may be necessary psychologically as well as physically. The reaffirmation of the commitment to their welfare which they may have, child-like, perceived as lacking in their own mothers may help them to begin the long climb back to physical and mental health.

An important advantage of in-patient treatment is that it is frequently the first opportunity anorectics have had for many years to make friends with people outside their own immediate family and their peers. When they are in hospital they are on neutral ground away from family, friends, school or job, and the expectations and demands of these. They are able to meet and talk to people from different backgrounds and of different ages. This is extremely necessary for girls who tend to come from over-involved families functioning within narrow limits. They are able to form their own opinions uninfluenced by parental criticism and to realise the problems people have in common. Many patients and parents see this as having been a most positive help.

Anorectics will also have to establish relationships with the nursing staff, some of whom are near them in age, and many of whom will have had personal experience of dieting. Some units prefer to have middle-aged nurses for this reason.

The nurses have the advantage of mutual support, and of understanding from the medical staff that they are likely to have some difficult and upsetting moments. Peter Dally has said that 'nursing a patient with anorexia nervosa is extremely wearing and tests to the utmost the understanding and emotional stability of the nurse. The strain imposed upon the nursing staff is considerable and it is essential that they are given adequate support. No doctor can manage any but the mildest case of anorexia nervosa without devoted co-operation from the whole of his team.'

How much more so for the mother. She has no devoted co-operation from anyone, no mutual understanding or support, painful emotional involvement and no time off. She is on duty 24 hours a day, seven days a week, often for years on end. She is the target for every kind of criticism, with no real opportunity to give her opinion on how the anorexia nervosa may have developed, and never under any circumstances is she given the benefit of the doubt.

Staff are well aware of the danger of the anorectic feeling that this is a passive experience, the weight gain being done to her rather than by her. They are careful to avoid taking her over and intensifying the feelings of dependence and helplessness which made the implications of puberty and of growing up so unbearable.

After the weight gain is progressing satisfactorily and the patient is up and about she may be hurt by the lessening amount of attention she is apparently receiving. This is deliberate, giving her time to absorb her increased under-standing of her illness and herself and to adjust mentally and physically to the additional weight and the inevitable change in her figure.

There are necessarily moments of rebellion and fear. A girl may not find it easy to substitute the control over others which has been sustained by her control over her eating with a genuine sense of her own identity, unsupported by manipu-lative manoeuvres. She is having to live through the part of her adolescence which she has missed at a fairly rapid rate. This will not always be happy or comfortable for her.

As her weight improves so does her general attitude. Hilde Bruch feels that not enough attention is paid to the dramatic effect of hunger on psychological functioning. Behaviour during the acute state of starvation or in long-lasting chronic starvation, reveals little about the underlying psychological factors. However, there are marked individual differences during these stages which must to a large extent be based on the pre-illness personality and the damaging effects of in-creased isolation. Some mothers feel that the starvation produces all the other symptoms, the presence of underlying psychological problems being grossly exaggerated. Anorectics tend to take the opposite view; most of them would welcome more and not less attention being paid to psychological problems.

Anorectics are so often told how privileged, good-looking, intelligent they are that they carry around with them a heavy and increasing burden of guilt. It is from these views that the punitive attitude towards them comes. How can girls as lucky as they are inflict upon themselves and their loving and caring families so much unnecessary suffering? They have so much to be thankful for, they have no reason to be so vin-dictive, so naughty, so spoilt and so tiresome.

They recognise all this but are genuinely unable to help themselves. They are often paralysed by fear, terrified of death, frightened and helpless. Parents live in constant dread of an anorectic daughter committing suicide.

There are occasional reports of patients who have repeatedly torn out drips or tubes from their throats so that eventually attempts to replace them have been abandoned and the patients allowed to die. Mothers are naturally afraid that this could happen to their daughters. Doctors normally feel that people with anorexia nervosa do not genuinely wish to die but that occasionally they are so severely emaciated, metabolically deranged and perceptually disturbed that they are unaware of their imminent death.

Two per cent do eventually commit suicide and at least 10 per cent of anorectics die from other causes related to the anorexia nervosa, including psycho-surgery. A patient who commits suicide when suffering from anorexia nervosa does so after many years of illness and despair. Early diagnosis and refeeding are of paramount importance.

Once an anorectic has achieved a target weight she will be allowed to get up, spending increasing amounts of time away from the hospital usually with one or more of the other patients. She may go shopping, to a cinema, to meet friends and generally begin to stand on her own feet again. Some mothers find this freedom worrying, having assumed that their daughter would spend all her time safely within the confines of the hospital.

They disapprove of her being taken to see X-certificate films or being allowed to travel on the Underground while she still looks so frail. The hospital is unfailingly irritated by the mother's concern but the conflict is one of degree. To a doctor who first saw her when she weighed 32kg (70lb) a girl of 42kg (91lb) looks much better. The mother who was accustomed to having a daughter of 57kg (126lb) before the onset of anorexia nervosa still feels she is dangerously thin. She is concerned about her physical safety, fearing that if she were to be attacked while wandering about or travelling she would not be able to defend herself. This is perfectly true.

The hospital is legally responsible for the girl's safety and welfare while she is an in-patient and must therefore take the view that the risk of psychological damage from continual incarceration in an institution is greater than the risk of physical danger outside it. One of the constant factors leading to and sustaining anorexia nervosa is a complete lack of self-confidence. It is essential for this to be regained and a degree of autonomy to be established.

Parents do not understand how extremely difficult it is for a girl, especially if she has been constantly ferried from place to place by her conscientious mother for most of her life, to make even the smallest expeditions alone. Only the known route, the already negotiated journey are safe, and only familiar people are trustworthy. The constant fear of the unknown, with its consequent isolation, extends to every aspect of normal daily life, denying them the opportunity to explore new territory, either physically or psychologically. A new bus route, a change of tube or train, can present appalling difficulties. The company of other people who have had or still have similar fears and will not laugh at their anxieties makes it easier to negotiate these hazards.

When she reaches an agreed weight the patient with anorexia nervosa will be allowed to have visitors. Mothers have different reactions to the visiting restrictions. Most consider them to be unkind. The lack of visiting is initially hard but it means that no emotional demands are made upon a patient. These may be unintentional, but the sight of the mother anxiously struggling in after a tedious journey, which she invariably mentions, worries her daughter. The mother is concerned if her daughter is not visibly blooming, tension accumulates and they start to bicker.

The separation gradually lowers the emotional temperature which is invariably heightened by the anorexia nervosa. Both mother and daughter are able to see one another in a kinder light. The mother fully realises that her daughter is seriously ill and is not simply a rebellious child, hell-bent on destroying herself and everyone with whom she lives. The daughter may realise that her mother is trying to perform a perfectly normal function of mothering – feeding a daughter who clearly needs it – and is not a hysterical tyrant.

The daughter may need to be separated from her family in order to see them in a new, more realistic, way. A mother does not always understand that the daughter's inability to be disloyal comes from an over-identification which is preventing her separating properly from her mother. Her development and individuation cannot continue until she can accept that she and her mother are two different people. The bond between them may need to be disconnected so that they may reconnect and communicate as individuals.

Once the girl has regained normal weight she will be allowed to go home for weekends to see how she feels about being discharged and returning to her family. A weight loss is an indicator of whether or not she is yet ready for this. The return is never easy either for the anorectic or her family. They will have realigned themselves and are worried about having to readjust once again. Both patient and family experience a feeling of dread mixed with jubilation.

There are likely to be difficult days ahead for them all. The siblings may be more apprehensive and hostile than the parents. This is a critical time. Mothers are convinced that if this could be handled differently it would be possible to reduce the number of readmissions.

It would be helpful for the mother to go to the hospital several times during the last weeks of her daughter's stay so that she can be with her daughter in an environment where her daughter feels more accepted than her mother. She needs to see exactly how much she can eat. Anorectics are notoriously untruthful about their eating, largely because of the fear of parental reaction. This would help mother and daughter not to humbug one another quite so much.

Doctors resist suggestions that a patient should be sent home with some form of diet sheet. They feel that this would be a retrograde step when she has altered her eating habits and behaviour and is now no different from anyone else. Mothers with practical experience of what actually happens when a daughter is discharged do not agree.

They are certain that it would be most helpful for both mother and daughter if they had some sort of progress chart detailing the expected food intake. This could be completed every day, perhaps for the first month, and shown to the doctor or social worker by both of them at out-patient visits. The routine of filling in a chart every day would impose a soothing discipline, and the failure to do so would also be an indication of how things are going. It would help the anorectic not to feel so abandoned by the people upon whom she has necessarily come to rely.

An Australian consultant has had very good results from a 'trust' system. Girls are free to come and go as they please, but must sleep and have their meals at the clinic. Only those who are unable to stand without fainting are kept in bed. The girls eat in the dining room with a dietician and nurse and a peer-group pressure develops in which the girls encourage one another. Many can go home within six weeks.

A girl who cannot go home may be able to stay with a friend or relation who lives near her family so that she may visit them, although never eating with them, and begin to be more independent and also maintain contact with them. Her stay with the friends or relations needs to be dependent on her eating what they provide.

It was suggested to me that families with an anorectic daughter might find it helpful to 'swap' daughters. They would understand the problems well and living with someone else's daughter might give them all useful insight.

6

Have You Met Her Mother?

> And last, the rending pain of re-enactment
> Of all that you have done and been; the shame
> Of motives late revealed, and the awareness
> Of things ill done and done to others' harm
> Which once you took for exercise of virtue.
>
> T. S. Eliot, 'Little Gidding'

Every mother's view of anorexia nervosa reflects her own conflicts. So it is that a mother who sees it as an attempt to dominate is one who feels dominated by one of her family and would like to reverse this. The mother who sees it as a refusal to grow up is perhaps herself unwilling to assume responsibility for all her own actions, tending to take refuge in ill-health to avoid any increase in responsibilities. The mother who sees it as a manifestation of a desperate longing for experience and freedom is one who feels trapped and frustrated, unable to find an escape.

If a mother can say to herself 'What do I think anorexia nervosa actually is?' and then answer herself from her guts rather than from other people's views and theories she will have taken the first vital step towards understanding.

The whirlwind effect of anorexia nervosa is such that once the process has started, after her daughter's withdrawal, it is unlikely to be easily reversed unless the family unit is stable and supportive.

The withdrawal of a daughter, especially in patients in the 11–14 age group, is seen as a reaction to the depression of her mother, leading to the daughter feeling abandoned and rejected at a time when she needs patient support to cope with the implications of puberty. Mothers tend to feel that any maternal depression follows the onset of the anorexia nervosa.

Anorexia nervosa in her daughter catches the mother unawares, dragging her relentlessly down into the Slough of Despond. She has no time to reach out for help, not realising that she must stand still in the middle of the whirlpool if she is not to carry everyone else with her. She feels sick with apprehension, trying not to see what is staring her in the face and being forced to do so at every mealtime. She is buffeted between misery and anger until she is punch-drunk, confused, clinging to rays of hope which have no substance and are too fragile to give her any support.

When persuasion, cajoling, shouting, bullying, pleading, tears, regular meals, irregular meals, meals in restaurants and meals in fields, arctic silences and bellowing rage have all failed to make her daughter eat she has a pervasive fear, a stark despair. Overpowering depression and anxiety set in, often before a doctor has been consulted. The mother cannot really believe that her daughter is trying to kill herself. She is in a constant panic, similar to that of a horrified, incredulous, parent watching a much loved child standing perilously poised on the edge of a cliff – near enough to be grabbed but threatening to jump if anyone attempts to do so.

The mother's terror and her tiredness, her disbelief and her duties, her guilt and her grief, her anger and her anguish all combine to defeat her so that she begins to live on two different levels. She has to be occupied, although increasingly less effectively, with the normal domestic trivia but most of her existence is immersed in a self-protective haze. She clutches the duster as if it were a life-line, drops it and lets it lie. She forgets the furniture, trying to remember anything that might provide a clue to her daughter's condition and the rejection of herself which it implies.

She becomes a distraught automaton, mentally over-active and physically under-active, restless and resentful. Her mind is never still, hunting, searching, apportioning blame, impatient with helpful and hurtful suggestions. She looks for causes. She is alert for criticism. What has she done, why has it happened, whose fault is it, how did it start, when will it end? What does she have to do today, why is there no food to eat in the house,'whose socks are these left lying about, how is she to cope, when will the children be home from school? How indeed is she to manage when she is so distracted, her daughter so defiant and the rest of her family so demanding?

But since the natural human condition is to adapt and so to survive she does somehow get from day to day. After a time even the most minute achievements come to represent major triumphs, so small do her days become and so narrow her aims.

Her days assume a pattern and routine, interspersed with waves of terror and bursts of crying. She cries everywhere, usually alone. She cries on the telephone and she cries in the bath. She cries when people notice her daughter's emaciation and comment on it. She cries when they do not. Her frequent bouts of sharp self-criticism, her shame and the exasperation of her family eventually have some effect and she regains her self-control.

She begins to resent other people's claims on her. She is now the only person in the world with such a dreadful problem. Why must she be bothered with other people's worries when her own are so much worse? So she protects herself, allowing isolation to envelop her until she is no longer able to be touched by anything outside her whirlpool.

The loneliness hurts her, the isolation suffocates her but she goes headlong on her downward path. She churns up memories, hunts out letters from her daughter, gazes at photographs of her looking well. She remembers incidents which might have upset her, regrets her own outbursts of anger over trivialities, wishes she had been more aware,

105

more loving, more perceptive, more communicative. She aches for a second chance.

Mothers vividly describe a time of black despair when a turning point seemed an impossibility. For nearly all mothers there is a turning point. It is when this is reached that a mother is able to begin to subject herself to a ruthless self-analysis which may help her to achieve a new stability, to stop running away emotionally.

She will be given no help, encouragement or guidelines as to how to begin this painful process. She starts her journey of self-understanding alone, knowing that she is likely to stumble across areas of hurt and humiliation she never knew existed.

At the beginning of her quest for enlightenment it is the isolation of which she is most conscious and most resentful. Isolation is defined as a neurotic defence mechanism, an irritating description for a woman to whom it is reality. She should greet any defence mechanism she is lucky enough to encounter with sighs of relief rather than with rage and rejection.

Isolation is necessary for self-analysis and for constructive reassessment. A mother needs the rest which it can give her if she allows it to, she needs to regather her forces. The more she fights it the longer it will last. She must stop feeling guilty if she is thinking rather than doing. She must not allow herself to be drained by other people's needs and demands. Above all she must refuse to allow herself to fall into the ridiculous but tempting role of the 'gallant little woman'.

She needs to take care of herself rather more, and of her family rather less. She has a great deal to do and needs all her resources to accomplish it. The alternative may be having a daughter who is chronically ill and unhappy and who will be her major care and concern for the rest of her life. Anorexia nervosa can become chronic, and once this happens no amount of soul-searching, of personal or professional analysis, of therapy, of abreaction, of separation, of medical or lay support is likely to reverse it. The future existence will be something approaching non-existence.

Her mind wanders most easily back to her daughter's early life, her often difficult or unusual pregnancy and birth, her own experiences throughout this time. Much more is now known about the psychopathology of spontaneous abortion and difficult pregnancies – she may consider the possibility that her problems were a measure of a deep-seated rejection of her husband.

She may think about the effect that she and *her* mother had on one another and consider the possibility of patterns being repeated. She may wonder if her own early separation from her mother has made it difficult to understand how children who live with their mother all the time could need or lack anything.

Anorexia nervosa inevitably appears to be a sign of acute maternal failure. The mother of an anorectic daughter comes to feel she has failed on so many different levels that she has nothing else to fear. Failure removes the fear of failure if a woman can see the freedom this gives her as a foundation for further development. She can allow herself to be angry, to be honest, to be less than perfect, to be ordinarily human.

There seems to be no obvious correlation between the length and severity of the anorexia nervosa and the intensity and duration of a mother's internal upheaval. They do not balance or counterbalance one another, nor do they run parallel. There is often a parallel between the need of mother and daughter to establish themselves as individuals.

Individuation was described by Jung as one of the tasks of middle age. Many mothers of anorectics are middle-aged. The mid-life crisis is not simply a term used by women's magazines to define the symbolic moment when a woman makes the agonising decision whether she should let her hair go grey or begin to dye it. It is a real experience, not unlike adolescence with its associated hormonal changes, and it occasionally seems to have the unfortunate or even tragic result that the roles of mother and daughter become re-versed. The daughter may take over the cooking and caring when she, rather than her mother, should be entering into a period of healthy rebellion and self-discovery. She realises too soon that the price of growing up is heavier than she had imagined.

Many mothers of anorectics had to shoulder responsi-bilities for other people, usually younger or handicapped siblings but also occasionally invalid mothers, at an age when they should have been exploring the full range of adolescent behaviour and establishing their own identities. Their uncon-scious expectation that their own daughters should be able to do the same makes no allowances for their daughter's tem-perament or the different circumstances of her upbringing.

Some mothers are aware of having a strong undercurrent of self-defence in their own personalities which manifests as passive aggression. Many feel that this stems from their inability to fight for themselves openly.

Many mothers describe the positive benefits they have obtained from their daughter's anorexia nervosa. It may sound surprising and even shocking that a mother can derive strength and self-confidence from her daughter's serious illness, but it is irrefutably true that for some women the whole unhappy experience and the traumas which come with it represent a catharsis.

Mothers find that they are able to communicate more easily with their family once the unnecessary barriers have been broken down. They have dropped their illusions about perfect motherhood, realising that living up to their own ideals may not be good for their family. Some see their existence as having been womb-like with both the limitations and the protection this involves. They have had to face the reality of possible death and have survived intact from the worst experience a mother can imagine – the lengthy, serious and possibly fatal illness of one of her children.

To outsiders the mother seems to be giving in, allowing

herself to be overwhelmed by events well within her control, unhealthy self-indulgent introspection. Surely the best thing to do with this problem is to ignore it. She has no need to allow that tiresome daughter of hers to run riot through the entire family, destroying herself and everyone else. The mother's guilt forces her to defend her daughter to outsiders while increasing her daughter's anger and resentment towards her. The daughter's debility and regression force her to become more dependent on her mother while increasing her anger and resentment towards her.

They are in the realms of the double bind, the pathological symbiotic hold, held to be among the expected childhood foundations of a psychosomatic adolescent illness. 'A child is put into a double bind', typically by its mother, by being made the object of incompatible, contradictory emotional demands in a situation from which there is no avenue of escape, and from which no other member of the family rescues the child by compensating for or correcting the mother's behaviour, or by elucidating it to the child.

This is the mother who says, 'If you do that again you'll be smacked' and does not smack after the sixth offence. This is the mother who laughs when she is angry. This is the mother who expects her small child to show her uncritical adoration, refusing to hold her child's hand when she is frightened because it might look silly or because she is herself too afraid to be able to tolerate fear in her child.

This is the mother whose love is dependent on being loved, whose ability to feel unappreciated is unbounded, whose fantasies of motherhood lead her to treat her child as though she is a member of a different species rather than the normal human being which she is. This is the mother who holds her child back while coaxing it forward, finding it hard to accept that children develop at different speeds. They can do so very well without her constant supervision and encouragement. This is the mother to whom the entirely sensible concept of 'observant neglect', known also as 'Breed 'em, feed 'em, and leave 'em be' is an anathema. Compensation takes on common sense and common humanity and wins.

Anorectics say, 'My mother was always boasting about me.' This may be a reaction to her mother's own childhood experiences which came from the unique need of English parents of a certain type and generation to write down and denigrate their children. How many women whose own daughters are now grown or growing up can remember cringing with embarrassment as they heard their mother' or father's ringing tones disparaging and apologising, apparently unaware that children, like foreigners and other disadvantaged classes, were not automatically stone deaf. 'Mine's the ugly one', 'Those are my little horrors over there. Aren't they ghastly, ha ha.' 'She's at that awkward age you know. Kinder not to look.' 'Whenever I bring this gawky girl anywhere she just droops about, picking her nose and scratching her bottom', 'We're praying she's got a brain.'

Where did this pathological terror of conceit and self-esteem come from? Why do some women feel so dreadfully unsure of their femininity that they take measures from their daughters' early childhood to prevent them enjoying their own? Why is it that even in this age of feminism and face-lifts it is still possible to find women who seem embarrassed by its existence?

The mother has to face the painful fact that anorexia nervosa is a manifestation of a deep early insecurity. At some stage in her daughter's early life something went wrong, and she does not have the necessary resources to carry her through the turbulent waters of adolescence. She is not certain enough of either her own strength or that of her parents to be able to make the traumatic break from childhood. There have always been daughters who needed to be near their mothers. The classic picture of a daughter caring for a domineering mother, now socially unacceptable, was as much a reflection of the daughter's need as of her mother's.

Many mothers either had difficult pregnancies or danger-

110

ous complicated births with their anorexic daughters. Some mothers were seriously ill during their pregnancies, some had a history of stillborn or handicapped children or had conceived shortly after the death of a sibling. Older mothers know that there is an increased risk of a deformed child born to a woman over 35. This contributes to a stressful pregnancy. Some anorectics have mothers in this age group.

Many older mothers had been successful career women with smooth-running, well-organised lives. They were unprepared for the disruptive effect of a baby and worse still a toddler. It may have been their first experience of the extreme exhaustion resulting from endless sleepless nights and of the unexpected feeling of isolation which being tied to a baby can bring. So much emphasis is placed on pregnancy and birth that many women fail to realise what lies ahead. It seems that sometimes a child has lost sight of herself in the need to make life tolerable by doing what was expected of her.

Difficulties in mothering were compounded by the fact that many mothers of anorectics have a vivid memory of having little or no physical contact with their own mothers. Very few of them felt valued. It is easy to blame previous generations, but this is a never-ending and pointless process. Did the 150th great grandmother come down from the tree backwards, thus conferring on her descendants a constitutional inability to face up to reality?

The mothers' experiences were frequently due to circumstances. Many women felt the war had had a disastrous effect on their childhood. Children were evacuated, finding themselves far from home and stable family life. Once the ties with a mother are broken, particularly if the child is too small to communicate by letter or is for some other reason unable to maintain contact, they may never be re-formed.

Maternal deprivation due to war, death, divorce or illness is a constant factor. The resulting insecurity of the mother may be reflected in that of her daughter. The daughter's ambivalent attitude to her mother reflects her understanding that she is luckier than her own mother was. She may feel that the love and attention she gets are not totally deserved. This can produce more guilt and anger than she can handle.

Many mothers of anorectics had early lives which were markedly more interesting and varied than those of their daughters. They have plenty to tell – adventures, dramatic or traumatic childhoods, tribulations and triumphs. This is good and necessary if it provides children with a wide base, an understanding of the infinite possibilities of life. However, a certain type of child feels annihilated by the realisation that she cannot do what her mother did. They see this as reflecting lack of character rather than circumstance. They may not understand that it is sometimes the reaction to the turbulence of their mothers' young lives which causes the slow tenor of their own.

There are many things a daughter may want to tell her mother. One of the most difficult to express is that she sees herself as dull. Over-compensation may be at the root of this. Mothers say that they wanted their daughter's childhood to be happy, to be different from their own. They wanted to break a pattern. It may be this wish which causes the pattern to continue.

Their thinking is inwards and backwards, whereas outwards and forward are really what are needed. Childhood is one stage in life, albeit the foundation, and should be regarded as such. Fantasy notions of the perfect childhood are usually based on early and often inaccurate impressions of other people's families and are very dangerous. Life for some begins but should never end with rocking horses and lullabies. No woman is going to make her children happy or sort out her own childhood problems by providing her children with everything she now thinks she missed.

'Understand the world you live in and be on terms with it,' wrote Rose Macaulay in *The Towers of Trebizond*. Mothers now in their 50s, 60s and 70s have had to be on terms with several different worlds, born during the First World War or the slump, growing up during and after the war. After this they had to readjust to the slower pace of peace in a period of rapid social change.

They never grudged the time given to their families but were themselves often frustrated. Girls suffering from anorexia nervosa nearly always regard their mothers as 'wet' despite the fact that many mothers have led interesting lives. This surprises outsiders who generally have a rather different impression, but the daughter is looking at proven behaviour and not at underlying temperament or appearances. They see their mothers as easily put upon, a soft touch, over-involved with other people and their troubles. Within the marriage they see lip-service as submission. They feel that their mothers' apparent inability to stand up for themselves means that they will not be able to defend their daughters should the need arise. They also fear that they themselves lack strength and resolve in the same way as their mothers.

Inevitably a mother thinks back to her adolescence, so different from that of her daughter. The mother of an anorectic is likely to have been brought up during a period of austerity, to have married before or during the sixties, thereby being confined to domestic life at a time when most women still accepted their husbands' interests as paramount. There were of course some people who could see that marriage and motherhood were not fulfilling for some women. Some of their daughters have developed anorexia nervosa.

The radical change in the attitudes of their contemporaries gave the mothers a feeling of missing out, of resentment at being apart from the popular tide of booming prosperity, pop music, mass-produced clothing, more for everyone. Attitudes towards sex were changing. Sex for the unmarried girl was made easier by the Pill, whereas for previous generations pre-marital sex was fraught with the danger of pregnancy.

It may be the backgrounds of so many mothers of anorectics which leads some professionals to look for the causes of anorexia nervosa in the fashionable and much discussed

113

fields of feminism. This may widen still further the speculation around anorexia nervosa.

Do girls dislike the prospect of becoming women because maturity in our society represents a loss of identity, an acceptance of limits to personal development? Is anorexia nervosa the feminists' revenge or is it a sign of an unacceptable female longing to be dependent at a time when women's independence is heavily stressed?

Why are so many women obsessed with their bodies? Why do they feel that an underdeveloped bust can lead to more personal fulfilment than a well-developed personality? Why do they feel so helpless and undervalued? Why do they feel it necessary to pretend that they want to be treated as men, when the majority want an absorbing interest which can be pursued at their own speed and to suit themselves. How many women really want to undertake the responsibility of keeping, educating and providing for their families from the age of 20 to 80, with little thanks and a barrage of abuse when they protest about changing the baby's nappy? A psychiatrist suggested to me that a girl may develop anorexia nervosa because when she was born her mother could not decide whether to love her or have a career. Why should they be thought mutually exclusive?

Why do competent, intelligent women feel they are reduced to cyphers unless they have a degree or a career? Women dread the question, 'What do you do?' They flounder, although their own common sense should tell them that they are living useful and fulfilling lives. Voluntary work is not allowed to count. It is almost necessary to have a degree in institutional management in order to fulfil yourself by handing out bowls of soup. All too often private charity equates with public insult even though the social services are incapable of giving all the help that is needed.

A mother whose children are leaving home or are in full-time education may wish she had had a training or career before her marriage to which she could now return. Many women had no burning ambition, no vocation, no encouragement. Those who were able and motivated enough generally got what they wanted. Is anorexia nervosa a disease of mediocrity rather than of originality, the fear of being ordinary rooted in a girl's personal observation of its frustrations and disadvantages?

It is never easy, even with outside encouragement, for a woman with no qualifications or experience to find an interesting occupation. Many women fear that their attempts to find a new lifestyle within the confines of their existing responsibilities may not be successful. Rejection sends them scuttling back to the oppressive safety of their own homes.

The mothers of anorectics generally lack the cutting edge and ruthlessness needed to project themselves successfully in a competitive world. They may therefore project their own hopes and ambitions on to their daughters. It may mean that energy which should be used positively is driven inwards, causing self-destruction and depression.

Anorectics are said to have remarkable *élan vital*, a passionate though suppressed love of life. They are felt to be people who are not able to realise their potential. This description applies equally to their mothers. They are seldom high-flyers. They are intelligent, competent women too unsure of themselves to live as productively as they could. Many are aware of this but do not know what to do about it.

Some mothers describe their anorectic daughter as 'so ambitious, so materialistic. It seems as though her masculine and feminine sides are out of balance.' They mean that they feel the logical and emotional sides of their daughters' personalities are out of balance, anorexia nervosa being an attempt to reconcile them. This is prompted by what they have read about hormone levels. Might it also be a perception of an internal conflict which is both more subtle and more fundamental than it appears?

When it is the masculine aspect of her daughter's character which concerns a mother she may also be rejecting the

115

masculine side of her own character which she keeps almost totally under control.

Not for nothing do nearly all the mothers of anorectics describe themselves as coming from a long line of strong women. Why so many of them are masquerading as shrinking violets has a great deal to do with their attitudes towards their husbands and the demands they make on their wives. It may be their way of removing themselves from competition in a male-dominated world, knowing that lessening dependence on a husband and some financial independence will be unacceptable.

What is the mother of a daughter with anorexia nervosa like? What sort of woman is she likely to be? How far can she be blamed for the onset of her daughter's illness? Is she guilty, misguided or unlucky?

She is usually middle-aged when the anorexia nervosa starts, although mothers' ages range from the middle 30s to the 80s. She is usually physically strong, conscientious, hardworking, loving, caring, manipulative, intelligent, competent and extremely stubborn. She lacks self-confidence and strong convictions, and is usually conventionally dressed. She tends to have illusions about being an all-providing earth-mother when she may have been too inhibited for this to have been reality. She is restless, anxious and possibly frustrated. She is most unlikely to be the typical Tory lady in a hat clamouring for the return of capital punishment. She is equally unlikely to spend her days campaigning for the CND. She is seldom daringly original and creative, although she may be artistic. She does not generally go through life on a permanent and dramatic high, leaving behind her a trail of emotional devastation and broken hearts. She is not always self-generating, generally giving of her best when she is reacting to a man.

Many of the mothers exhibit a very distinct attitude towards authority, leading them to show their children a good-humoured tolerance which may have more to do with inertia than with the painful disciplines of love. It may indicate an ability to disengage from the difficult and from any complicated emotional contact, coupled with a feeling of helplessness when faced with the obstacle of a stronger will than their own.

This is the mother who may be a floating voter. She may have the vaguely liberal ideas and ideals of anyone whose housekeeping money does not depend on her husband being more likely to be kept in work by one government than by another. This is a mother who may not regard established authority as automatically right, being inclined to the more cynical view that rules are there to prevent anarchy rather than because they necessarily have an intrinsic moral worth.

A mother hears that she has either been too strict or too permissive with her anorectic daughter, in spite of the fact that her other children seem able to survive her methods. Mothers have regrets about incidents in their daughters' childhoods which they feel might have been handled better, although given this child's temperament and her mother's reaction to it there was probably no alternative. There are very few women who cannot see the mistakes they made and the problems they have led to.

Many mothers lose their self-confidence and are temporarily unable to be rational. There is a stage when they see the anorexia nervosa as a massive rejection by their daughters, a carefully calculated and highly effective revenge. As she sees her anorectic daughter getting thinner and iller, as she sees her other children 'acting out', and as the relationship with her husband declines into an abyss of quarrelling and mutual blame, interspersed with bouts of temporary mutual support engendered by panic, the mother feels total degradation and overwhelming despair.

This is the moment when more than anything else in the world she needs another mother in the same situation to talk to. She is helped by being able to discuss her feelings and experiences with someone who understands. The strain on her family may be alleviated. She definitely does not need anyone who deals with anorexia nervosa in a professional capacity. It is essential that no breath of criticism from someone without personal experience of the problem should inhibit the free exchange of painful and distressing feelings or the description of ways in which mothers come to terms with anorexia nervosa and their role in helping their daughters to recover.

Mothers feel constantly criticised and blamed for unwitting and unintentional mistakes. Criticising the upbringing of other people's children is a favourite parental sport. It does not involve the onus of proof and has the added thrill of the danger of sudden reversal when the protagonist's own child is unexpectedly found wanting. Friends and relations 'could have told her . . .' Why did they not? She suddenly finds herself faced with other people's unpalatable views on her maternal incompetence and – far more hurtful – on her daughter's character.

The mother has to extract from the comments the jealous, the irrelevant and the purely speculative and be honest with herself about any criticism which she knows is fair, constructive and well intentioned.

She must continue to see her friends, sidestepping discussion about and criticism of her daughter by talking about something else. She would be well advised to keep any sharp retorts and pertinent comments on her friends' children firmly to herself, realising that they feel threatened by anorexia nervosa in the child of a close friend.

She has got to stop feeling sorry for herself. Many mothers feel they are having a far worse time than any other mother. This is thoroughly silly.

There are thousands of mothers whose whole lives are devoted to the care of children who have been mentally or physically handicapped since birth and are without hope of any kind. They have the constant and harrowing worry of what will happen to their children when they die or cannot look after them any longer. They are the recipients of an

118

unexpectedly large amount of unkindness. Unbelievable as it may seem, a number of parents with thalidomide or other obviously damaged children have been accused of having deliberately caused this damage in order to make money out of it. Their children are often in constant pain, or suffering from the side-effects of drugs which may be used to try to help them. They are nearly always unable to be mobile and independent.

The situation of an anorectic and her family is nothing like as bad as this. It is a serious illness but a great many anorectics continue to be independent even when they are severely emaciated. Nor are their mothers confined to their homes. It is much better if they are not. Anorexia nervosa is sometimes unbearably difficult because of its negative effect. Anorectics do not appear to want or be able to extract any enjoyment whatever from their lives and are often totally un-cooperative with anyone trying to help them. This is why mothers feel so desperate, hopeless and defensive.

As the mother lives with the illness and encounters the various professionals dealing with her daughter, she may find herself for the first time thinking about the nature of modern parenting. Parents in our society are in a hopeless position. They have little actual or legal control over their children once they are 16. They may not choose their schools or hospitals unless they can pay handsomely for the privilege, nor are they able to have any say in what goes on in them.

They have to stand back and see their daughters being covertly encouraged to embark on sexual intercourse before they are emotionally ready, by being offered a birth-control pill many of them forget to take. If their daughters become pregnant (early pregnancy – sign of distressed family) they are faced with the alternatives of the daughter possibly sustaining emotional damage from an abortion or with having to look after the baby while she continues with her education. If a child becomes a drug addict their own family doctor considers it to be his duty to protect the child's interest (i.e.

119

keep to himself its self-destructive habits) until the problem is beyond his control. The parents are then expected to assume responsibility both for their child's welfare and for its condition when, had they known what was happening earlier, they might have been able to obtain specialised help at a time when there was hope of a real cure.

The function of parents is to pick up the pieces and pay. For some of this they are themselves to blame. Schools in particular have great difficulty in providing the discipline necessary for both education and stability if the parents do not provide discipline at home. Parental problems are partly the result of the cult of the individual, which has considerable disadvantages when the help of the community is required.

I am temperamentally disinclined to look for Reds under either my own or anyone else's bed nor do I find it easy to talk rationally about the forces of evil. Nevertheless one is forced to see subversion and evil intent as real forces when so many parents who should know better allow people whose intentions are not always clear to interfere between them and their children. Until families assume responsibility for their own children they will have nobody but themselves to blame if things go wrong. The insidious effect of a welfare state is the assumption by far too many people that if something is wrong with one of their children someone else should deal with it.

The boundaries need tightening within society as a whole as well as within some families. Why do we allow ourselves to be undermined to such an extent that we are uncertain how to deal with problems in our families, uncertain of our own ability to know what is best for them? By this I do not mean that anyone within a family who requests or requires professional help should be denied it. I mean that if families could only once more assume that they know what is best for their children a great deal of trouble could be avoided.

7

Husbands and Fathers

> A man of sense only trifles with women, plays with
> them, humours and flatters them . . . but he neither
> consults them about, or trusts them with, serious
> matters.

The Earl of Chesterfield, *Letter to his Son*, 1748

A mother may spend some time thinking about contemporary marriage, her expectations of it and her willingness to
contribute to her own. The divorce rate in anorectic families
is low, implying to psychiatrists that conflicts are kept below
the surface. Anorexia nervosa causes a family crisis which
may lead to the breakdown of an already shaky marriage. It
nearly always affects the marriage and the partners' feelings
about one another. The changes are seldom for the better,
the conflicts often being left unresolved while the bonds of
love and companionship between husband and wife are
broken.

Hilde Bruch observes that the mothers are submissive to
their husbands in many details and yet do not truly respect
them. It appears that some mothers of anorectics have unconsciously chosen to marry men upon whom they could
consider themselves to have conferred a benefit. They may
feel later that they deliberately denied themselves the opportunity to grow and develop emotionally and psychologically,
removing from their lives the possibility of success and
acceptance as well as of failure and rejection.

There is often a marked disparity between the backgrounds of husband and wife, more noticeably between the two sets of grandparents. This may be racial, regional, economic, educational; occasionally there is a marked difference in age, but the most obvious discrepancy is of social class. A wife may experience difficulties if her husband has succeeded in establishing himself in the strata to which he wants to belong.

A man with a working-class background may regard a wife who works, or wishes to do so, as reflecting his inability to support her. He may be unable to see why she finds the way of life he has achieved limiting. He feels he has done all that can be expected in providing for her and his children materially, and resents her need to expand other areas of her life. If his mother was out at work so that he had to come home to an empty house he quite reasonably wants to feel that his children do not have to do this.

Background confirms identity and provides security so that uncertain adolescents can see a pattern which is strong enough either to revolt against or to conform to. When this is nebulous or disparate a child is placed in the dilemma of which way to jump. The daughter who resembles her father is most likely to suffer from anorexia nervosa. She may have always identified with him, having been told all her life that she is just like him either physically or temperamentally. She feels that any criticism exuding from her mother also includes her.

She is in the intolerable position of identifying with the disadvantaged parent. She resents him and hates her mother for creating this situation in the first place. It would be unfair to say that some mothers may have seduced their daughters but so is the way in which many of them have allowed their children to despise their fathers.

Both parents may have been guilty of hurting and annoying one another through this daughter who is sensitive to the needs of both and torn apart by them, the whole process wrapped in layers of good intentions and responsible parenting.

A girl whose parents were happily married and sympathetic to each other's values and points of view would be unlikely to develop anorexia nervosa. 'Happy' marriage is hard to define, so perhaps 'adult' marriage is a more accurate description.

An adult marriage is one in which both partners are mutually involved, supportive and caring while at the same time able to allow one another freedom to function as individuals without being either jealous of or threatened by the other's independence of thought or action. Their individual strengths combine to give their children support and stability, unhampered by the too intense concentration on them which an unsatisfactory marriage can produce.

Damage can be caused, including anorexia nervosa, when the parents are so intensely involved with one another that they neglect or disregard their children.

The doormat wife is thought to be a relatively recent phenomenon, a male-induced reaction to the Married Women's Property Act and to feminism. This is not true. The intrinsic nature of many women has always made it difficult for them to reconcile the emotional satisfaction gained from loving and caring with a realistic approach to their own identities and interests. Héloïse, a brilliant and reluctantly successful woman wrote to her lover, Peter Abélard, in the twelfth century: 'If only your love had less confidence in me, my dear, so that you would be more concerned on my behalf. But, as it is, the more I have made you feel secure in me, the more I have to bear of your neglect.'

Some mothers find it difficult to have a balanced relationship with their husbands, feeling unappreciated and misunderstood. They see their husbands as ambitious, selfish men who only pay lip-service to women's rights. The hard truth remains that able, energetic women with intelligent well-adjusted husbands have always been able to work without spoiling their marriages. An adolescent may see restriction and undervaluing as part of her female, adult life.

Few mothers would prefer to have remained unmarried, feeling that happy marriage is the ideal state for a woman, the best environment for the rearing and bearing of children. They may not be able to see that irksome restrictions may be of their own making, blaming their husbands and children for imposing boundaries which no pressure could make them heed if they really wanted to escape.

Distance lends enchantment to moments in everyone's life but not usually to the marriages of an anorectic's parents. Some mothers feel that they went into marriages which had less to do with love and acceptance of their husband as himself, more with what he represented as an escape from their families. Some say that their husband was the first person to whom they ever really mattered. Some mothers started their marriages feeling guilty about leaving mothers to whom they had been tied, having been made to feel that they should never leave them.

It was not the fashion, nor would it have been compatible with their mutual need for emotional security, for the anorectic's parents to discuss the underlying motives and compensations in their marriage. Both husband and wife were more strongly influenced by their backgrounds than they would have been prepared to admit at the time. For many anorectics there arises during their emergence into puberty a serious internal conflict in trying to reconcile the two sides of their personalities represented by their mother and father.

Some mothers had fathers who died when they were young or who were killed in the war. They have dream fathers, marvellous, kind, brave, glamorous whose memory they worship. Their relationships with other men are almost bound to be disappointing and to disappoint. Many have vivid memories of their fathers' physical presence.

Some mothers had no brothers, so their fathers projected upon them the ambitions they would have had for their sons. Nearly all the mothers whose fathers were alive during their childhood or adolescence have a distinct attitude to men resulting from their upbringing.

They see men as rare, special and threatening. They saw at an early age that women could manage very well without them. Their own mothers brought up their children, ran their houses, worked and survived without their husbands' constant presence and help. Their daughters did not understand that their mothers were often lonely and frustrated and were afraid of resuming normal married life with husbands with whom they had lost constant contact and who would try to take over the authoritarian role of head of the household which many of them were thoroughly enjoying.

The ending of the war, or the return from the colonies, meant that girls saw their own mothers being relegated to a purely domestic sphere. The fathers picked up the threads of their paternal role with children who had grown away from them. They did not always want to accept that their wives had managed without them.

For some mothers the war had opened new horizons and opportunities. They never really recovered from being told they were of no more use. A few women were so devastated by this that they were unable to come to terms with post-war life. Their impressionable daughters took upon themselves the burden of fulfilling their mothers' dreams. When their own children were born they were torn by the contrasting needs of both their mother and their eventually anorectic daughter. They were unable to reconcile their two different responsibilities. Girls with anorexia nervosa resent their mothers spending time with people outside their immediate family. They feel threatened by the prospect of someone else's needs being greater than their own.

At the beginning of the anorexia nervosa there are no holds barred in their encounters with their husbands, a great deal of venom and resentment is released by both sides. As the illness progresses this may change to mutual concern – two impotent parents instead of one, occasionally leading to a closer bond between partners. Daughters take upon themselves the role of marriage-mender. Once this happens it becomes incumbent upon both them and their parents to maintain the new-found harmony. The instability of its foundations makes a fragile liaison which can be easily upset. The whole family become more and more enmeshed in order to avoid the possibility of still worse traumas.

During moments of reflection, mothers considering their feelings about their husbands, find it hard to be either objective or fair. Mothers report that their husbands give them no help or support with their anorectic daughter. When asked if this is really true many are surprised to find that they have made it impossible for their husbands to help. Some husbands may have opted out but others have been pushed out.

Some mothers of anorectics feel themselves to be overprotected and over-controlled by their husbands. It seems that a mother's control over her daughter reflects more nearly the controlling factor within her own marriage than a resurgence of adolescent conflict about the control exerted over her by her own mother.

It is almost impossible for the recently divorced mother of an anorectic daughter to take a properly objective look at her own husband or other people's. I have made an assessment of the fathers and their role which is based on other people's comments and writing, coloured by my own experience and observation.

The father of a daughter with anorexia nervosa may be very ashamed of her illness, seeing it as a personal failure and occasionally convinced that it is a deliberate attempt to humiliate and annoy him. Intense worry may alternate with intense rage.

Some fathers see the anorexia nervosa as a sign that his women are trying to irritate him and distract him from his own affairs. He may be prepared to put up with some feminine frailty from his wife but he expects more than this annoyance from the daughter whom he was confident would reward his efforts to provide her with an expensive education or constant attention by being a credit to him.

'Absolutely typical' is his initial reaction. This progresses through a series of hostile and unhelpful phases, interspersed with bouts of highly emotional concern, until it culminates in obvious rejection. This includes the rejection of the possibility of any form of psychiatric illness within his own family, rejection of medical advice, rejection of any suggestion that he might have in any way contributed to the onset of anorexia nervosa, a severe if not total rejection of his daughter's need for his support.

Other fathers are able to take the illness less personally, although never completely calmly. They are sensible enough to realise that although both their wives and daughters need some support from them there should be limits to their involvement. If both father and mother can retain some degree of detachment from this predicament there is a much better chance of a satisfactory outcome.

Anorectics generally feel undervalued by their fathers, although outsiders may have the impression that they were over-valued. They feel their fathers never made them appreciate the pleasures of being female, by encouraging them to mature into attractive and independent women. There is a real problem when a father does not want his daughter to grow up, either because it makes him feel old or because he prefers to treat all women as little girls and is not doing too well with his wife.

Incest is a fashionable psycho-sexual problem, increasingly discussed, but it is not usually sex but conversation and adult companionship which are missing in an anorectic girl's contact with her father. The girls often feel intellectually slighted and treated as children even when they have high academic and other attainments. This may be exaggerated by girls who have no brothers and have been to single-sex schools, so having no opportunity to form non-sexual attachments with men other than their father.

127

Many fathers had as children to bear the full focus of family expectations. They may be only sons or ones who have for some reason been regarded as 'special' within their family, often having no one with whom to share the strain of over-expectation. Many have never had to fight in order to establish their superiority. The habit of responsibility is so ingrained that any abrogation of it within their own families imposes a heavy burden of guilt.

Anorectics often come from fairly large families, few are only children. The fathers often wanted large families without any idea what this entailed. The function of children is to occupy their parents, to irritate, to make demands upon them, to enchant and to exasperate. A man who was brought up without interfering siblings, who never had a game disrupted, his belongings rifled through, or his room invaded by other people's small friends can find the effect of being constantly in a family unexpectedly overpowering.

What is so sad is that the fathers of anorectics love them so much and are so distressed by their illness that they cannot see it objectively. They are ashamed of anything in their families that might discredit them. They reject the daughter upon whom they have imposed the greatest demands at a time when she most needs their support and understanding.

Many fathers have put so much effort and time into furthering their ambitions that they have little energy left over for their children. They will do anything possible for them, apart from facing the anorexia nervosa constructively, giving them anything and everything apart from time and easy affection. 'No normal father has a conversation with his own children,' said one of them. Many anorectic daughters know that this is what their fathers feel.

They are proud, as all fathers are, of their daughter's invariably attractive appearance. A daughter may be made conscious of this before she is capable of comprehending the difference between paternal and sexual love. She may find her father embarrassingly intense in his attentions to her, and is aware and afraid of her mother's jealousy. The difficulties he experiences about physical contact somehow make this worse.

He may have had to reject his own mother's constant attention in order to survive and this makes him uncertain of limits which other men understand. This is not the sort of father into whose arms an unhappy or tearful little girl could throw herself for comfort or reassurance. He may be awkward, inclined to find the possibility of casual arousal too threatening to be permissible with anyone other than his wife.

There may be little physical contact between father and daughter. Anorectics who make suicide attempts when they are with their fathers are demonstrating a need to be closer to their fathers, to be cared for by them.

Many fathers are tense. Many suffer from migraine and various forms of largely psychosomatic stomach disorders. These may affect the eating habits of the rest of the family.

If a father finds that his daughter's attitude to him is changing, becoming hostile and withdrawn with occasional bouts of intense attachment, and can take the time and trouble to give her more attention, taking a greater interest in her appearance and amusements than in her academic success, a great deal of unhappiness might be averted.

The anorectic's relationship with her father changes as the dieting progresses. It is largely governed by his reaction to her anorexia nervosa. There are some fathers and also some mothers who will defend almost literally to the death their daughter's right to starve herself. A father may cling on to the illness, not wanting it cured because it is the only time he has really felt needed.

A father who does this in spite of his wife's continuing and intensified efforts to make her daughter eat finds that he and his daughter can become more closely allied in the struggle against their mutual enemy – the mother. The daughter

129

clings relentlessly to her father – once more the little girl he wants her to be – and soon they are stuck in their newly acquired roles. The father is St George, the mother is the Dragon.

A mother can be very jealous of her daughter when this happens. She bitterly resents the new alliance and feels betrayed. She perceives her authority is being undermined and feels excluded and censured. She is panic-stricken at her inability to persuade her daughter to eat. She, and the siblings, begrudge the time her daughter and husband spend together and the new clothes and presents he buys in a futile but understandable attempt to make her happy.

This is a very unhappy situation, all the worse for being transitory. The father nearly always gives up the unequal struggle. His wife is faced with a daughter who is not only very ill but also hostile. She is desperately hurt by her father abandoning his new-found role as her protector and blames her mother for this.

The mother needs her husband's support but she must in turn support him. 'Mother loves us, mother cares, mother will wheedle what we want out of that wonderful, understanding, sadistic ogre – father.' Mother would help everyone if she could stop wheedling and allow the father to distribute money and other forms of help to his children according to what they both think is fair and to what he can reasonably afford. He may not find it any easier than she has done to deny his sick daughter extra benefits but he must be consistent and fair, bearing in mind that in anorexia nervosa uncertainty is a great deal worse than injustice.

WHAT CAN A HUSBAND AND FATHER DO TO HELP?

He can help by taking over control of the financial affairs, becoming the only parent to whom children can appeal for money, setting and sticking to rigid rules about the amount each child is allowed. His anorectic daughter will not be helped by being given more than her siblings. As always, it is vital that she is not treated as 'special'.

He can help by taking his wife out more. Many husbands seem to spend several years while their daughter is ill sitting at home complaining how bored and neglected they are. Distraction and amusement are therapeutic for both husband and wife. He might take his wife out alone once a week.

He can help by arranging that any business entertaining he has to do is either done out in restaurants or with help provided by him without complaint. His wife may find it impossible to cope with this for a long time – at least until his daughter is eating normally.

He can help by ticking off his daughter if she is rude and offensive to her mother. It is not good for her to be allowed to deepen any existing rift between her parents. The mother must do the same.

He can help by not referring to his intellectual superiority – his wife feels hopeless and inadequate as it is. He will not help by ganging up with his daughter against his wife – treating his wife as half-witted and his daughter as intellectually gifted.

Husband and wife can help one another by not discussing the 'peculiar' behaviour and characteristics of one another's families.

He can help by not being hostile or aggressive to his daughter's doctor or contradicting his advice and treatment. Fathers have greater difficulty than mothers in accepting anorexia nervosa, finding mental illness most upsetting.

He can help by buying his wife some new clothes and paying her some attention instead of sulking.

He can help by being more authoritarian, leaving his wife to do the mothering.

HOW CAN HE HELP HIS DAUGHTER?

He can help her by spending time with her, by being firm with her, by not wanting to keep her as a little girl.

He can help by taking her out. He may be ashamed of taking out a girl who is emaciated and bedraggled but she needs to feel valued by a man, and her father may be the only one available.

He can help by showing an interest in whatever she is doing, without telling her what a splendid future she will have if she really makes a go of it. He must not let her know that he is disappointed by her performance. He must accept her as she is.

He can help by not telling her how much nicer she looks now that she is thin. Girls have occasionally been driven into anorexia nervosa by a father's constant and cruel criticism of their appearance and figure.

He can help by not wandering around the house in an undressed state. Anorectics, and other daughters, may be embarrassed and upset. He can also help by not canoodling with his new wife or girl friend in front of her. He can however help by showing physical affection and love to her mother.

He can help his daughter by not making snide remarks about all his efforts having been for nothing. He must try not to be too hurt and angry.

He must not be tempted to help her behind her mother's and siblings' backs, thinking that everyone else is too hard on her and he alone understands. Mothers feel it is important to be cross about uneaten meals because the daughter needs to know that her mother cares enough to notice. Patients complain that if they eat alone with their father he never seems to notice whether they eat or not. The poor man is usually trying to be tactful and not upset his daughter by paying too much attention to what is going on.

132

He can help by not blaming her for any trouble in her parents' marriage or any 'acting out' by her siblings.

He can help her by finding new interests and outlets for himself. She badly needs to respect her father so that she may begin to rely on him. It is helpful for his daughter to gradually become less dependent on her mother by relating more to her father.

He can help her by encouraging her to expand her horizons by, say, learning to drive and by helping her to do so.

He can do most to help by treating her exactly as he would expect to treat any other normal, intelligent, responsible and attractive young woman.

8

Acceptance

> Blank acceptance never leads to a solution. At best, it
> leads to a standstill and is heavily paid for in the next
> generation.
>
> Jung, 'Memories, Dreams, Reflections'

Around a mother whose daughter has anorexia nervosa there
hovers constantly the spectre of the spoilt child. A spoilt
child is recognised as one who has been spoilt by her parents,
i.e. denied the loving discipline and care which give security.
Many girls who develop anorexia nervosa have had since
early childhood a quality of being 'born spoilt', of requiring
more than other children, both emotionally and materially.

Experienced child workers see this as a reaction to maternal depression or distraction leading to a genuine lack of
adequate attention and mothering. This illustrates the way in
which environment is thought to dominate heredity, denying acknowledgement of a child's intrinsic character. Any
mother knows perfectly well that children's characters remain remarkably constant through all the vicissitudes life
provides. She is able to accept them as they are rather than
imagining that the more prickly aspects of their characters
can be radically altered.

Acceptance on many different levels is the key to sur-
mounting anorexia nervosa for the patient and her family.
Both the illness and the temperament of those who develop it
need to be understood in order to be accepted. This accept-

ance leads to more positive attitudes, making the illness easier for the anorectic and her family.

The girl who develops anorexia nervosa is intelligent, perceptive, hypersensitive, materialistic, stubborn and loving. She has pathologically low self-esteem, in perpetual conflict with her ambitions and her poor self-image.

Her level of intelligence is not always as high as her academic success may indicate. She works hard to achieve and is too conscientious to keep her efforts within reasonable limits. The amount of time she spends on her work means that as examinations approach she is forced to withdraw from her friends and outside activities to concentrate on her studies. She may be a girl for whom the glittering prizes are tantalisingly close at hand but forever out of reach. She may be a late developer, steaming ahead academically while clinging to childish emotional patterns of behaviour, the one masking the other.

There used to be a term, long since out of use, which perfectly describes the anorectic. 'A sensitive' was a pretty, intelligent girl with an unfortunate knack of finding the most difficult way of doing things. She had an over-developed capacity for being hurt, each hurt increasing her obvious vulnerability.

She was introverted, thoughtful, sometimes chronically lonely, with an inordinate fear of death and dying coupled with an enhanced perception of, and rapport with, the supernatural, and with a psychic sensitivity. This increased her natural anxiety, making her too aware for her own good of the unsaid and the unseen. She was uncompromising and idealistic, and therefore often disappointed both in herself and in the people she loved.

She was deeply aware of and affected by pain and suffering. Such awareness can only increase in an age in which international tension and the continuing build-up of nuclear weapons make everyone aware of the possibility of annihilation. The fear of what lies ahead is as relevant to an anorectic's illness as anything in her childhood.

She was artistic, impressionable, shy, finding it difficult to express her feelings easily. Her frustration led her to defend herself with an intense anger which took other people un-awares. She was likely to over-react to criticism so that it was often easier for her to carry her worries alone than to discuss them with others. Trusting anyone was both painful and difficult for her.

She was someone who found life troublesome at the best of times; nowadays even more so, for in addition to her own intrinsic difficulties she may have to bear the burden of the possibly unreal expectations of her parents, school and con-temporaries.

False expectations lie at the core of anorexia nervosa. There are those of the anorectic herself so far as her success and future are concerned. There is the confusing expectation that children can remain 'childlike' when they are constantly exposed to an adult world through films, television, comics, magazines. These may induce a false maturity unsupported by matching emotional development.

There are the expectations of her siblings that she will continue in her role as the 'good' one, which considerably reduces pressure on them, leaving them free to express themselves in a less inhibited way. There are the expecta-tions of her school or college that she will be a credit to them, emerging from their hands a well-behaved, academically successful, balanced member of society. In reality she may have been tightly controlling a longing to kick over the traces.

She has to face the expectations of her peers and family as to how young, intelligent, pretty girls should behave. She feels driven to succeed in every way; to be attractive, aca-demic, athletic, artistic, assured. She must be careful about her appearance and able to deal with sexual advances. Girls with anorexia nervosa are attractive and a retreat into an asexual child-like state can be protective.

The modern teenage girl may feel she is expected to reject

the traditional female role, which may be all she wants. A recent survey carried out by a Sunday newspaper found that an unexpectedly high proportion of girls in a London day school, well known for its exceptionally high academic success rate, still see marriage and children as their main aim.

She may have the burden of the expectations of her parents, especially her father, that she will be a credit to them, bolstering their wavering self-esteem by conspicuous successes. She may also have less obvious expectations imposed; for instance she may be cast into the role of a son by a father disappointed that all his children are girls. She may feel that she is meant to compensate for her mother's supposedly missed opportunities by pursuing the career and liberated lifestyle which were not available to her.

She may be burdened by the expectation that she must compensate for a dead sibling, although parents seldom if ever consider this her role. A sensitive child who hears her parents talking about a dead child and realises the grief they still feel may try to replace the dead sibling in some way. She may feel that she is a replacement and must therefore make herself perfect and lovable. If she was born near or after the death of a much loved mother of either of her parents, and whom she resembles, unexpected assumptions may be present that she will replace the grandparent and ultimately care for her parents.

Unless she has a strong enough personality to resist the inroads made by the expectations of both other people and herself, she will have to find a defence in order to survive. Anorectics have a negative attitude, stemming from a pervading feeling of helplessness. Even after they have been cured, many of them years later still give the impression of having an emotional wall around them, a fear of being hurt, a holding back from the risks of living.

Girls who develop anorexia nervosa are afraid of the sound of quarrelling. They dislike noise. They seldom go to large parties or discos with their friends and this naturally cuts them off from their contemporaries. Mothers say teen-age parties and other social occasions are frightening to a girl who is shy or self-conscious.

One mother described the anorectic's extreme suscepti-bility to atmosphere when she said, 'She only comes to life when she is in the right atmosphere for her, with people she trusts. It is really tragic to see the way she chatters and laughs when she is in the right surroundings. People misjudge her, thinking her characterless and dull, whereas she has a mar-vellous sense of humour and is a terrific goer once she gets started.'

In addition to the discomfort and fear which come with anorexia nervosa the patients suffer greatly from the dislike, resentment and irritation which the illness arouses in other people. They are accused of bringing the trouble upon them-selves in order to attract attention, to disrupt their family, to avoid facing up to reality, to get out of their responsibilities, to avoid growing up, of being selfish and ungrateful, of being mad, or being dangerous to their contemporaries who may copy their self-destructive behaviour. Anorexia nervosa is not a deliberately self-induced illness. This is certain. It is however an illness from which a girl can help herself and be helped by others to recover.

The dislike and fear which ascetism and self-denial have always aroused are illustrated in John Donne's letter of 1608 in which he defends monks: 'they owed the world no more since they consumed none of her sweetness nor begot others to burden her.' The hostility aroused by anorexia nervosa cannot, however, be dismissed as the result of a materialistic society seeing this apparent rejection of its values as an attempt to undermine its foundations. It may be that the slimming success of the anorectic represents to some a major achievement in an area in which many women and men fail, so that some degree of jealousy is involved in the hostility.

Anorectics would see all the arguments from a different point of view, answering criticism with criticism, fear with fear, emphasising that anorexia nervosa is a complicated illness in which it is often impossible to distinguish between cause and effect.

They know that their dieting was never consciously intended to lead to anorexia nervosa. All women diet at some time and any woman who has done so knows how quickly it becomes an obsession. Women who normally spend as little time as possible thinking about food find themselves aching with anticipation for half a grapefruit, drooling over a plate of spinach with a semi-congealed poached egg on top. They know very well the frantic dash to the bathroom scales in the morning, the disappointment if there is no weight loss, the delight if one more pound has disappeared. Anorectics describe an imp in their heads which urges them not to eat the meal they badly want. This is no more than an exaggeration of the conscience from which all slimmers suffer when faced with some tempting delicacy.

The need to be babied is so much part of the anorectic condition that mothers are forced to ask themselves why this should be so. Some accept that an adolescent would only want this sort of attention if she had missed out in early childhood. The birth of a sibling causes a variety of reactions in a small child. The shock of being supplanted can cause emotional difficulties. However careful mothers are to ensure that their child or children do not feel neglected, the baby's constant demands, which are both absorbing and exhausting, can cause a brother or sister to feel left out. Some children feel rage and resentment towards the new baby. Others are delighted with the sibling but intensely angry with their mother for treacherously providing a rival for her affections.

Many mothers of anorectics are warm and loving but there are others who experience real difficulties in cuddling and hugging their children, being unable to show much warmth in spite of the love they feel. Some women just do not like small babies. As the child grows up, the minimal physical contact which existed in childhood dwindles to practically none at all.

Even when the mother is demonstrative and loving there may still be problems. Many of the parents are unused to showing one another any affection in front of their children, so busy are they demonstrating their independence to and from one another. The children, observing the distance which their parents maintain from one another, realise this might happen to them. They are not secure because they can see that the giving of love is arbitrary and if they offend a parent their love might be removed. They perceive that love can be conditional.

When a friend's son said to me, 'Anorexia nervosa all boils down to a lack of love', I was shaken and ashamed. He seemed so sure, so calmly certain he was right. It is hard to understand how a child who had been properly loved in the way she needed could have developed anorexia nervosa. Surely such a determined turning away from life must stem from a deep sense of rejection in earliest childhood. Or does it come from her mother's inability to evince the 'appropriate response' of 'good enough mothering'?

The mother accepts that the lines of communication between her and her daughter have been broken or temporarily disconnected. There are in many families members who are not on one another's wave length, who cannot either in childhood or when grown up understand and communicate with one another. This is sad but it is fact, and underlines the great weakness of psychiatry – theory is fine but when it comes up against the reality of human nature it may take a nasty fall. The best that can be hoped for is that age, experience and increasing mutual tolerance lead eventually to a degree of understanding and acceptance between people who are naturally at odds with one another.

Anorexia nervosa has the striking advantage for an unhappy daughter of being free and requiring no props. A girl causes the maximum disruption without the misery of explanation. As she sees her weight slipping lower and lower she experiences a feeling of power, increased self-respect, the realisation that for the first time in her life she is in control. This is her reward for her self-denial and discomfort.

Control is a major factor in anorexia nervosa. The anorectic sees her control over her own body as her only defence against being controlled by other people. Anorectics feel hopelessly vulnerable, unable to control their own destiny. A sufferer may feel that in reinforcing the dominant side of her personality her weaker aspects may be annihilated or absorbed so that she is 'in one piece'.

When considering control in anorexia nervosa as it relates to present-day adolescents, a paradox appears. Most adolescents are less controlled than their parents were but anorectics always talk about the over-control exerted upon them by their parents. This must be partly due to their appalling lack of self-respect which makes it impossible for them to respect others and to accept control from them.

There is something wrong with parental control as experienced by an anorectic girl. Some mothers over-control their children because individuality and self-expression are intolerable. Other mothers have little or no control over their children, thereby failing to provide the security which all children need before they can become independent.

Does the anorectic need to control her family because she feels its organisation is haywire? Is it because she feels inferior to, and undermined by, a sibling or parent and asserts herself in this way as the only means to survive? Is she trying to rouse her mother to establish a strong enough control for her to relinquish her own once the family structure is stable enough to give her the support she needs? Is it the result of an over-developed sense of responsibility? Is she trying to repay hurt with hurt?

Is her control directed towards preventing others from coercing her into growing up and taking responsibility for which she is unready? Is she resisting her parents' attempts to push her into performing well, so covering them with reflected glory? Does she feel like this because her perception of what may happen to young adults nowadays is distorted or because it is accurate?

Acceptance of her daughter's needs and character can be difficult for a mother. 'I love my daughter but I don't like her very much', say some mothers. The anorectic feels the same about her mother. It is hard for people involved in a power struggle to like one another. This requires mutual understanding and respect, tolerance and good communication.

It is not always clear whether a daughter is really being either under- or over-controlled, or whether her inability to break through the shell of her own personality is responsible for the apparently distorted control.

So we see a girl whose emotions are under abnormally tight control and who has been simmering and repressing her feelings since infancy or early childhood. Many parents knew their daughter was frustrated. They had hoped each new stage of development, walking, talking, learning to read would make her happier. Everyone who works or lives with an anorectic is aware of her pent-up anger. The intensity of her feelings is matched by her difficulty in expressing them.

The quality of goodness referred to in writing concerning anorexia nervosa is more complex than mere good behaviour. Some mothers say their anorectic daughters were abnormally quiet, never crying for a feed. Others say their daughters were restless and unhappy as babies, the 'goodness' only showing itself as they grew older. Others have no idea what the talk of 'goodness' is about, as their daughters were lively and naughty at home until the onset of anorexia nervosa. They were usually good at school. 'Good' means that they never argued with their parents, accepting what they were told without question, they never refused to go to bed, they ate what was put in front of them, they never swore at visitors, they never wrote on the walls with felt pens, they never picked a fight with their siblings, they never lost their tempers, they always did their prep. They never showed their feelings because this might upset their mother so everything that worried them or made them angry was bottled up. When they needed to let off steam they did not know how to do it.

Some anorectics were totally incurious. Lack of curiosity, before and during anorexia nervosa, illustrates difficulties in communicating and in being involved with other people.

Girls with anorexia nervosa suffer from distorted perception, genuinely seeing themselves as enormously fat even when skeletally thin. Their delusions about their size are outside their control and are largely responsible for the misunderstanding and intolerance the illness arouses.

The inability to see may merit more attention. Some success has been claimed by practitioners who correct the visual distortion by standing a patient with anorexia nervosa in front of a mirror and projecting around her an outline of the size she perceives herself to be. There appears to be a connection between people with migraine and those with anorexia nervosa. The only conclusion I came to after four years with my anorectic daughter was that anorexia nervosa resembles a prolonged build-up to a migraine without the release an actual migraine would bring.

Should our society accept responsibility for the increase of anorexia nervosa? Anorectics are convinced that they have been influenced dangerously by the enormous emphasis on slimming and its importance for success. Psychiatrists dismiss this influence, while admitting its existence, ascribing its development to deep-seated psychological problems which manifest in an inordinate need to be thin. They acknowledge that some girls have a hypothalamic trigger which enables them to continue losing weight when others are unable to do so.

Is the media to blame for the increased incidence of anorexia nervosa? Slimming magazines, aids and diet books increase in number and popularity. Health clubs, exercise classes, health farms and weight-control organisations abound. Little effort is made to check on a potential client's health even when she is obviously emaciated. It is regrettable that medical certificates are not the rule before a strenuous course of exercising or dieting is embarked on. Hopefully organisations who are without scruples about removing money from girls who palpably do not need any help in losing weight will develop a more responsible attitude.

A great deal of money is being made from slimming – £200 million in Great Britain last year. If the slimming industry was forced to be less or non profit-making the incidence of anorexia nervosa might well decline.

The media can be blamed for glamorising anorexia nervosa which is in reality a dreary, miserable and unglamorous illness. Articles appear stressing the risks of permanent physical illness which can come from anorexia nervosa but there is undeniably an element of mystery and exciting danger in some of them.

Society reinforces the illness both with condemnatory attitudes and with fake ideas about social standing. Families come from a wide variety of backgrounds. It is wrong to describe all of them as affluent. They are affluent only in the sense that all in Western society are affluent as opposed to the poverty of the Third World.

Parents sometimes accept that they applied too much pressure to perform. Some children are sent to school far too young. Nursery school education which enables women to work may mean that some children are over-stimulated and pushed to compete when they should be developing their own personalities within their family. They need to establish themselves as individuals in order to cope with growing up in a society which imposes harsh educational and social demands on children. There is something seriously wrong with a system in which mothers' competition about their children's progress allows little room for individual development.

Children in private education are more at risk because the process is so expensive that it is sometimes a question of value for money rather than of value to the child. Competitive examinations may start at the age of five or less, reaching hysteria point when children are sitting for their secondary or public schools.

Schools in the private sector lay great emphasis on the academic achievements of able children. 'She must be brilliant to have got in here', 'We only take the cream', 'She's a high-flyer.' Something appears to go wrong during the next five or six years since 99 per cent of adolescents who emerge from these establishments are in various grades of average. Above average, below average, well-above average, average, a good average – all with average as the key word. Truly, the number of brilliant people in any country, let alone any specific academic year, is small.

The mother has to accept herself. Her first reaction is 'What have I done to deserve this?', her second 'It's all my fault', thirdly, 'It has nothing to do with me. She decided to have anorexia nervosa.' Should she see herself as evil genius or victim?

No one deserves to have anorexia nervosa and no one should accept the blame. A mother may realise that she allowed conditions to develop in which anorexia nervosa could flourish. She may accept that she ignored warning signs because she hoped it would go away or because she or her husband were afraid or ashamed of having an anorectic daughter.

A mother will have to accept that a great deal of criticism will be directed at her, most of it behind her back. She will also accept that the attitude taken towards her by anyone trying to help her daughter is likely to be hostile. No one will tell her why this is so or on what grounds the prejudice is based.

This is not imagination. I have heard professionals discussing among themselves the mothers of daughters with anorexia nervosa. They are described in a number of highly critical ways, but most usually as malign and malevolent.

Malevolent, meaning literally 'wishing evil to others', is a most serious word to use about a mother. The inference is that a mother wishes to do her daughter such harm that she induces in her an illness or state of mind which may lead eventually to her death. This is an assertion which would not stand up to even minimal cross-examination in a court of law.

Furthermore, it appears that psychiatrists use words which are imprinted on the minds of a not always well-informed audience, causing them to behave subsequently in ways which add considerably to the distress of both the patient and her mother. Careless talk does not only cost lives in time of war.

The description which seems to best fit most mothers of girls with anorexia nervosa was sent to me by a friend who does not have an anorectic daughter but may have some insight into its problems as her own mother describes her as an 'anorectic manqué'. By this her mother means that her daughter has the right temperament and background but comes from the wrong generation.

'Most of the screwed-up kids I know have unstern, un-demanding, pleasant, sometimes rather dull or boring, naive and frequently perplexed mothers. These mothers always seem to come to grief with the one of their children who is stronger-willed than the average and who really wants des-perately to love and revere that parent. Instead, the child finds him or herself despising the parent for her weakness. The child will do almost anything to try to goad that parent into some harsh retaliatory action that will stop and suppress the child and put it in its place where it knows (better than the parent) it ought to be. I understand very well the feelings of children who are strong-willed and intelligent and who set themselves rigorous standards, finding themselves despising their parents and not respecting them (not hate, not indiffer-ence) against their own will and therefore seeking to hurt them.'

Many mothers of anorectics are well aware that their

daughters despise them. They react by sliding into apathy, absenting themselves from real contact with their daughters.

Some mothers accept and understand their curiously ineffective, although deep, concern about their anorectic daughters. This comes with the apathy, the giving up of the struggle. I was aware of this in myself and could not understand why I held back when I should have spoken out, why I was not always prepared to make more than a minimal effort, either physically or mentally. Anorexia nervosa demoralises a mother rapidly but I can see now that what was also involved was a subtle rejection, a refusal to engage, coming from intense and prolonged anger.

When the anger evaporated, with the help of a healing service, I had the energy to do what I should have done years ago – to face it honestly and engage in a battle with my daughter which I intended to win. I do not think any severe case of anorexia nervosa will ever be permanently cured until the mother, or occasionally a mother substitute, is able to regard the struggle between herself and her daughter as one between good and evil. By this I mean 'good' as healthy survival and 'evil' as self-destruction. The daughter's lack of self-esteem which is fundamental to her condition reflects a lack in her mother's self-image. Its recovery depends on her seeing that her mother is unafraid and unaffected by what is going on.

How much responsibility should a mother accept for her daughter's anorexia nervosa? 'It's all my fault' is ridiculous, discounting all the other influences to which a child is subject – father, siblings, extended family, friends, school, peers. It also more seriously discounts the personality of the patient, the reactions to her of other people and the effect that these have on her.

I have naturally considered the factors which led to my daughter's anorexia nervosa. Permanent marital conflict of a dreary and confusing variety must have affected her. Parental conflict may be stimulating to the partners when it is one facet of deep emotional involvement, its constancy being accepted by the children of the marriage and providing a certain sort of stability. Ours was deadening rather than dynamic, both for ourselves and at least one of our children. There were two brick walls, two battling egos fighting for supremacy, two people too afraid of the consequences of defeat to allow the other even temporary victories. An immature marriage which by its nature made individual growth and development within its framework impossible.

I was always gullible, over-reacting to the smallest aches and pains. Coming from a family of 'good-doers' with a vigorous enthusiasm for life I was initially disconcerted to find myself with a baby who was frail, constantly sick and showed no inclination whatever to thrive. I had, I think, a rather childish view of children's happiness, while recognising that adversity strengthens character, that challenges successfully met give more self-confidence than anything else.

I am asked whether anorexia nervosa has changed my life; if I feel enlarged or destroyed. Looking back on it now I can see that for me it was simply another stage in life. I regret only that it caused all my children to suffer in various different ways. I do not feel emotionally crippled by it as other mothers sometimes say they are. Neither do I feel that it has strengthened or radically altered me. I am more detached but less able to be involved. I have more self-control but less self-confidence, more tolerance but less patience. I am perhaps less easily amused but also less inclined to make a joke of things which I should take seriously. I am less impulsive but more determined, less tense but more lazy. I am much more resistant to pressure but am still inclined to react emotionally when I should use my head.

Anorexia nervosa was not as difficult for me to understand and accept as it was for any of the other mothers I have met and talked to. I first encountered it when a school friend

148

developed it at the age of 13. Since then I have known a series of sufferers, some who made a complete recovery and some for whom the illness became either mildly or seriously chronic. In every case some member of the anorectic's family benefited from the condition. Some mothers find they benefit from the continuation of the anorexia nervosa.

The greatest problem with which doctors are faced is that of collusion. Collusion occurs when the anorexia nervosa is maintained either by the sufferer and/or any other member or members of her family because of the benefit they obtain from its existence. The benefit most commonly mentioned is that of a family being united by their mutual concern for the patient. As long as she is ill their rivalries, their realisable and unrealisable ambitions, their hopes and disappointments can all go into abeyance.

Even when doctors are clear in their own minds about the possibility and type of collusion in a family, they have the utmost difficulty in explaining it or pointing it out in such a way that the unconscious pressures which are being applied to a patient in order to prolong her illness for whatever purpose are changed.

Sometimes the patient turns the illness to her own advantage, sometimes to one or both parents or a sibling. It may cater to a need of an anorectic's husband, or in the case of much older patients to a need of their children. This does not mean that it was deliberately induced by anyone involved, merely that in the creation of new problems existing ones may be removed or altered. This book is about the mother's role in anorexia nervosa, so it is the possible advantages to the mother which must be considered.

A woman may gain a feeling of importance. She is the centre of attention, the recipient of sympathy and interest, although you would have to exist normally in a state of mindless boredom for the rewards to justify the distress. This is a real life drama. A mother may feel able to reassume the maternal role which she could not replace satisfactorily. She

149

has a renewed sense of purpose and may be able once again to see her daughter as a child rather than as a rival. Some women have difficulty in accepting a daughter's sexuality and development into an attractive and fecund woman.

It may be hard for a mother to accept that one of the functions of anorexia nervosa is sometimes to reunite husband and wife in a mutual concern for their daughter. The anorectic is in a terrible position, seeing that as she recovers her parents will start to fight. She is too frightened to start eating, probably too frightened to swallow.

The mother's natural concentration on her anorectic daughter may enable her to sidestep difficulties with her other children. She can use it as an excuse. She refuses to go out with her husband (can't leave her alone), to move house (too unsettling), to make love (too tired and upset), to produce proper regular meals (food is a nightmare).

It may help her to avoid looking after a dependent elderly relative. It may be possible for a mother to turn the situation to her own advantage. It may be necessary for her to do so.

She may never really know whether she used the illness as an excuse to escape from her marriage. Did she destroy her marriage because it was the only way she could see of putting a stop to any further damage? Or does she do so because it is the only way she can morally justify escaping from a personally destructive marriage? She has no guarantee, however strongly she feels, that it was the quality of the marriage which precipitated her daughter's development of anorexia nervosa.

Emphasis on strengthening the parental relationship is essentially right since security is fundamental to recovery. A daughter may gain a false and temporary support from a marriage which is being held together by her illness and the collusion by all the members of her family who have a need for it to continue.

If a mother realises that a false alliance is only delaying the day when reality has to be faced she may decide that the only answer is divorce. She must be certain that this is the only way in which peace and stability will be obtained for her anorectic daughter, her other children, her husband and herself. She is taking upon herself a serious responsibility. She has to accept that if her daughter's condition worsens she will have no one but herself to blame. She risks undermining her daughter's stability to a point where it may be impossible to re-establish. She will alienate and enrage her husband at the moment when her daughter most needs his support.

She will be in emotional, domestic and possibly financial disarray. She is certain to upset her other children. Worse still, it will be necessary for her to be in constant contact with her ex-husband for at least the next two years. Furthermore, it will be wrong for her to embark on anything other than a very discreet love affair of her own.

She will soon find out that the wheels of the law grind exceedingly slow. From the time she and her husband separate until the divorce is final there will be a most difficult period of uncertainty, tension and distress for everyone. There is no tenable argument for a trial separation. Certainty is a priority. Until both parents have achieved some kind of domestic stability it is likely that her daughter's condition will worsen, possibly quite dramatically.

Nor is the future going to be easy for the mother. She will have to manage everything alone, making sure her children do not feel guilty, making enormous efforts to enjoy life without being drawn into an emotional relationship which she probably both needs and wants. She has to avoid being unkind about her ex-husband and avoid trying to hurt or irritate him by refusing to let him see his daughter. She needs to be with her children as much as possible since even a distraught mother is better than nothing.

The effects of a divorce vary considerably. The uncertainty, the tensions, the rows leading up to a separation may do more damage than the divorce itself. Parental behaviour after a divorce needs to be considerably better than before it. Parents owe it to their children to make every effort to make realistic and workable arrangements about visiting and so on.

By the time the divorce is obtained both parents and their anorectic daughter are at a low ebb. A new stability can be achieved and must be before the anorectic's condition can improve. Her mother needs to reassume control, consolidate, reassemble and rebuild a life for them all. The family need to care for one another before further development is possible for any of them.

Parents must release one another. A parent may continue to control the other through the anorectic daughter, may use her as a bargaining point or as a scapegoat.

I do not think that daughters who develop anorexia nervosa have a greater degree of concern than other girls about their parents' marriage breaking down; it is traumatic and devastating for all children. They do, though, have an unusual capacity for carrying other people's burdens and for feeling guilty and so may unwittingly place themselves in the position of a scapegoat.

The anorectic's inhibitions and fear about sex, and her understandable insecurity, mean that it would probably be dangerous for her mother to embark on a second marriage or permanent liaison until her daughter is much better. Any child of divorced parents can be badly upset by seeing either of her parents in bed with a new partner. Nor will a girl be helped by being in the middle of a possibly tempestuous parental love affair or by having to adjust to step-parents and their children. Mothers know that a few years of celibacy for them are infinitely preferable to a lifetime of anorexia nervosa for the daughter.

It may take a long time before a daughter feels secure enough to face the strain and fear of getting better. Life needs to be as normal as possible. A girl who sees her father mooning over his girl friend and her mother moaning about money may wonder if there is much point in being an adult.

A mother has to accept that her daughter is capable of making her own decisions, her own mistakes. She accepts that her daughter's unwillingness to conform to parents' ideas and ideals may be as much a criticism of the system as of them.

She may have to accept opinions from her daughter which she and the father may have induced themselves, i.e. guilt about starving children in the Third World. Parents who habitually tell their children they must eat up everything because of the starving children in the Third World are furious when the children refuse to eat on the grounds of feeling guilty because they have so much more than the children in the Third World.

A mother may accept that she has over-protected her daughter. The over-protective mother is regarded as causing enormous harm. A mother is unlikely to over-protect a child unless she feels she needs extra protection because she is highly sensitive and obviously vulnerable. As the crime rate rises, the brutal assault and murder of young children continue unchecked, as the number of young children killed in road accidents increases, the instincts of mothers to protect their children will quite rightly also increase. A change of attitude on the part of responsible mothers will only occur when a responsible society makes this possible.

The over-protective mother is one who does not allow her child enough mental and physical freedom for it to be able to develop in its own way and at its own pace, but school teachers, psychiatrists and social workers who regard protective mothers as a definite problem are simply going to have to find a way round it.

Mothers will continue to follow their instincts, knowing that it is the failure to do so which is likely to cause the greatest problems. They are inundated with literature and advice which undermine their confidence, encouraging them to depend on others instead of relying upon their own common sense. The high-flyer, the gifted child, the late developer, the hyperactive child, the educationally subnormal are perfectly ordinary human beings of varying abilities and tastes, all requiring the appropriate response which too many mothers are afraid to give them.

Mothers of girls with anorexia nervosa are thought to over-protect their daughters. By the time they see a doctor they probably are doing so. It is the outward and visible signs of anorexia nervosa which lead to so much trouble. Anorectics look terrible, thin, gaunt, grey in the face, ill and frail. Mothers are horrified when they hear people in shops muttering, 'What a pathetic sight', 'She looks half dead', 'Her mother shouldn't take her out in that state.' Naturally they feel and are protective about their emaciated daughter, naturally they fly to her defence far too often, so weakening her ability to defend herself.

Julian of Norwich's description of Mary's feelings for Jesus is applicable to most mothers' feelings towards their children. 'She was so oned to him in love that the greatness of her love was cause of the greatness of her pain. . . . For as much as she loved him more than any other, even so her pain surpassed all others. For ever the higher, the mightier and the sweeter that the love is, the more sorrow it is to the lover to see that body that he loves in pain.' The pain in anorexia nervosa is emotional, physical, spiritual and mental.

A mother may find it difficult to accept her daughter's need for emotional support outside her immediate family. Indeed the lack of this may be a pre-condition of her anorexia nervosa. Her daughter needs to break through the charmed circle of family life, making friends with different points of view and different standards. The support may be from a close girl friend, an older woman, usually an aunt, grandmother or godmother, or from a boy friend or therapist. It is pointless to feel jealous or inadequate. It is obvious that any girl who has felt so inescapably controlled by her parents that she has become seriously ill needs the opportunity to make a life outside her family. Accepting or rejecting family traditions and values is a normal part of teenage development to which the increasing dependence of the anorectic puts a halt.

A mother has to accept herself. This may be painful but she cannot accept her daughter until she accepts herself.

Anorexia nervosa makes mothers extremely angry. They are horrified to find within themselves a capacity for hatred, loathing and rejection. 'I never thought I could hate another human being so much', 'I pray daily for her death so that she may have some peace and so may we.' 'She was so weak, so repulsive I had a strong primitive urge to throw her on a dung heap to die like the runt of the litter', 'When I touched her she shrank from me as if I was evil yet when she clung to me pathetically I wanted to throw her as far away from me as possible.' 'She has destroyed our family, my husband and I loathe one another, the other children don't want to come home and when they are here they bicker all the time. They resent anything we do with her and then blame us for not making enough effort to understand her. If we try to do things together she ruins them.' 'She is so sweet to my friends that they think I imagine what goes on', 'She has become another person, she is no longer recognisable. This creature is no longer my daughter.'

Mothers have to come to terms with an anger which is contrary to their image of themselves, of normal mother-hood, their upbringing and their usual behaviour. They find themselves indulging in refinements of cruelty – like the mother who slowly squeezed an orange over her daughter's clean hair and down on to her spotless white dress, knowing quite well that the anorectic's obsession with cleanliness would make this seem the grossest violation.

Physical violence is occasionally demonstrated by both mother and daughter. This may start from a mother being determined to prevent her daughter leaving the room before she has eaten or to stop her going to the lavatory to vomit her food up. The mother who regularly threw her daughter into a bath after meals and sat on top of her for an hour was doing her best to stop this happening. Unfortunately initial violent encounter can turn into a habit, becoming the only emotional level on which contact continues between mother and daughter. There is a great deal of frustration in anorexia nervosa. A situation can develop in which a mother may find the physical violence stimulating and satisfying – even the worst difficulties of her present predicament seem preferable to the dreadful vacuum which would stretch ahead if these were resolved.

So the mother accepts herself. The daughters see their mothers as women who have devoted themselves to an image of wives and mothers which ignores their own needs, ruling out the possibility of being prime minister and/or a demon lover. They feel it is the mothers' views of themselves which limits them so, this in turn curtailing the development of the whole family. When mothers feel their daughters despise them and the daughters feel undervalued, the aggression and violence, physical and emotional, between them is likely to increase.

A mother may accept that her sexual attitudes have frightened her daughter. 'Girls develop anorexia nervosa because their mothers are sexually repressed and inhibited.' True or false? Insult or accurate observation? The comment warrants definition.

Is a mother inhibited and repressed in that she has told her daughter that sex is dirty and disgusting, pointless except as a passport to a kitchen sink? Or is she inhibited because she feels current sexual mores for young girls may be physically and psychologically damaging? Does she feel that sexual freedom may lead a girl into a bondage which will prevent her making the sure foundations for her future which are necessary at a time when marriage is undergoing rapid change and adjustment? Does she discourage her daughter's interest in it?

Does it matter what doctors think about a mother's sexuality? It matters when it unfairly affects attitudes towards the mother and influences the treatment of her daughter. What can a mother do about the psychiatric *idée fixe* short of murmuring 'Come up and see me sometime'? Nothing.

Does a girl reject sex because she has had an unhappy experience, because she was sexually aware too young, because she was frightened by hearing her parents making love, or because she was exposed to or touched by a man, often a relation or family friend, and was too frightened of being accused of lying or of being blamed to tell her parents?

Some mothers have found sex unrewarding, often reflecting a general lack of pleasure. Some may be jealous of an attractive daughter. Occasionally mothers refer to a daughter as 'such a tart'. After a time a pretty daughter may of her own accord or with her mother's subtle encouragement withdraw from an increasingly hazardous area.

Mothers may have difficulty in understanding the pressures adolescent girls may be under. We were not exposed to the erotic stimulation of films, newspapers, television. We were largely protected from the demands and expectations of sex until we were old enough to make our own decisions. Sex was for grown-ups, not for schoolgirls. We did not have to make decisions which might have been counter to our best interests because opportunity was limited, supervision strict.

On the other hand, adolescents today are kinder to one another than we were, able to be friends and companions in a way which would have been difficult for us. They are more loyal and protective of one another's interests. Unfortunately this can involve covering up self-destructive behaviour, the earlier discovery of which would lead to timely intervention.

The rising divorce rate adds to the problems. Girls no longer see marriage as safe, instead it is fraught with danger. It means that girls who are approaching adulthood may be burdened with mothers who are once again free and hopeful.

A girl may be distressed to see her father with a wife or girl friend nearer her age than his. Teenage girls are inclined to fantasise about their mother's sex life; seeing her with a man who is not their father may be disturbing.

After an anorectic has recovered she may start bingeing, accompanied by a period of compulsive sex. She may feel used and dirty. Starvation reduces libido and makes response less likely. This may create further problems. A girl may be afraid of sex because she fears it may trigger off uncontrollable impulses.

Mothers feel that it may be the emphasis on sex as the great liberator which can lead an adolescent to withdraw into the safety of her family if she has been hurt or disappointed in an early sexual encounter. Secondary patients may begin to starve or to binge or vomit after an unhappy sexual experience sometimes leading to an abortion. Mothers of older girls may reject the possibility of their daughters being sexually active. A mother may be 'quite sure nothing *happens*' although she is happy to say that her daughter is living with a man in a one-bedroom flat containing a double bed.

Mothers may not respond with an enthusiastic 'Yes' when asked by a psychiatrist whether the whole family spend time together discussing sex. Most would see no point in doing so, regarding sex as a private and intimate experience, although prepared to answer questions frankly.

Anorectic families have a low divorce rate but it seems that some parental sexual relationships are minimal and unsatisfactory. A marriage may have lasted for 15 or 20 years but if physical contact has not been maintained even in the simplest way by people who have not had the habit of touching and tenderness towards others from childhood, it is possible that the need and urgency of sexual intercourse during the first few years of marriage may not have developed into the satisfying recognition of mutual need which gives strength and support. Anorexia nervosa may bring to the surface dissatisfactions and resentments which were accepted when the family unit was stable.

Most people recognise their own qualities in others. It is here that the paradox must lie. A woman with a normally passionate and sensual temperament who should ostensibly be able to deal with the subject may find herself in a difficult position. Even the mildest discussion can make it clear to a daughter who is nervous, inhibited and in need of guidance that her mother's experience is rather wider, or far more limited, than might be expected.

A mother may not feel it sensible to discuss with her daughter the difference between technically successful sexual intercourse and strong happy lovemaking, but she may feel that not to do so is wrong and therefore avoids the subject altogether. She may inadvertently give the wrong impression – to mention the value of a sense of humour is more likely to give her horrified daughter an unedifying picture of her mother ripping off her clothes with shrieks of giggles than to describe the lighthearted depth of understanding and pleasure which can exist between two people who are at ease with one another and confident in themselves.

'Love maketh all things straight' but it also carries with it pain and responsibility. A woman who functions on a fairly intense level herself may feel that it would be wrong and damaging to encourage her daughter to set out on an emotional voyage with which she may not be physically or mentally strong enough to cope. Girls nowadays are made to feel that the absence of what is euphemistically described as a full and happy sex life in some way reflects on their attractions and femininity. They may feel instinctively that to be fondled by a spotty 16-year-old may not be the erotic delight they have been led to suppose. They want to develop their own lives before they become part of someone else's. This leads us back to the depressed housebound mother whose lifestyle her daughter does not wish to copy, and so rejects puberty.

Mothers are disconcerted to find the normal pains and pleasures of growing up categorised as psycho-sexual conflicts. They inevitably see the rejection of puberty as a rejection of themselves. A mother who has tried to give her daughter a warm and loving home will be hurt by this apparent wish to avoid her fate, feeling that many years of effort and care have been in vain.

Mothers may have a jaundiced view of easily available abortions, knowing from their own obstetric experiences that even a spontaneous miscarriage leaves a legacy of depression and guilt. Adolescents are fed with two conflicting messages. The idealisation of childhood and motherhood as the greatest joy and most fulfilling experience available to women conflicts with free abortion, which allows women to opt out of this, if temporarily inconvenient, by killing the baby.

Mothers' feelings about adolescent sexual permissiveness are based on evidence that increasing incidence of adolescent disturbance relates to increasingly permissive attitudes and open encouragement from people who represent authority to children and who choose to see themselves as part of the stabilising force of society. Some mothers think that it is their failure to provide their daughters with firm guidelines which makes them so frightened. Have we let our daughters down by accepting values with which we do not agree?

There do not appear to be any serious studies of the incidence of anorexia nervosa in the daughters of prostitutes or of women whose bodies are involved in their livelihood. It is therefore fair to assume that a woman who has a realistic approach to her body may not feel guilty about it, seeing it as an integral part of her personality rather than dissociating from it so that she sees it as an object, and that her daughter might also feel the same about her own. It may be that acceptance of the great variety of man's sexual needs and behaviour is lacking in some women whose daughters develop anorexia nervosa.

And so a mother learns acceptance. There are a number of

things which do not have to be accepted. The blank accept-ance which may underlie anorexia nervosa has to be turned into positive understanding and the willingness to accept a change of attitude.

There are some commonly held points of view which a mother does *not* have to accept. It is in everybody's interest that she does not do so.

She does not have to accept anger, helplessness, despair and total frustration as a way of life.

She does not have to learn to live only one day at a time or to accept that she is losing control of her own life.

She does not have to accept that using logic, bribery, force or punishment are merely a waste of energy and emotion. Logic and punishment may be of little use but bribery and the force of determination are not.

She does not have to accept that she needs professional help to bring up her daughter. In many cases she is far better off without it and so is her daughter. If she does have pro-fessional help she does not have to accept that she has failed any more than she would if she was unable to set her daughter's broken leg.

She does not have to feel overwhelmed by the irony and injustice of it, but she does have to keep a sense of pro-portion, remembering that time heals, although not always by itself, and that each generation of parents makes and carries its own particular crosses.

She does not have to accept that her daughter is clever, self-centred and selfish but she does need to understand that anorexia nervosa will make her appear so.

She does not have to bury her goals and hopes for the future for herself although she may have to accept that her daughter is not going to be able to live her dreams for her.

She does not have to accept that adversity is necessarily strengthening, self-enlightening and enlarging for herself, her family or her daughter. Some women feel that they and their daughters have emerged from the experience with more compassion and tolerance than they had before it. Others find that their own difficulties have made them very much tougher and less tolerant with other people's.

She does not have to accept anything she is unable to accept, neither guilt, neglect, over-indulgence, help from other people, blame from her family, insults from her daughter, advice from people who have no idea what they are talking about. She will accept as much as she is able to and discard the rest. She needs only to accept her daughter as herself, anorexia nervosa as an illness and time as something that passes.

9

Reality

We may not be taken up and transported to our journey's end but must travel thither on foot, traversing the whole distance of the narrow way.

Clement of Alexandria

'I would have done anything if only I had realised my daughter was getting anorexia nervosa, but I did not know how to begin. No one could tell me what to do.'

Parents of anorectics may read this at various stages of the illness and for different reasons. Some think their daughter may be developing anorexia nervosa and want to know how to be sure. Can it be reversed in the early stages and if so, how? Other parents have a daughter who appears to be dying in front of them and are panic-stricken, desperate for guidance. Some have daughters who are teetering on the brink of recovery and are uncertain how to help them. There are parents whose daughter's anorexia nervosa is now chronic. They are concerned about her future, anxious to make life tolerable for her and the rest of their family.

What can a mother do if she thinks her daughter may be getting anorexia nervosa? She can weigh her so that she has a guideline for increasing weight loss. She can make sure she is having regular well-balanced meals with the rest of the family. She can encourage her to go out and see her friends.

If the daughter is working obsessively her mother can try to stop her doing so. She can ask her daughter's school for a homework timetable showing how long she should spend on each subject. If she is taking more than twice the time suggested her mother must talk to her form mistress or headmistress about it. She may not be able to cope with the work, either because it is too difficult for her and she needs extra help or tuition, or because she is using excessive studying as an excuse to withdraw from her family.

The daughter may feel that she will only gain her parents' approval and love by showing them she is doing her best to live up to their expectations. Her fear of letting them down may be inhibiting her efforts to work productively. She needs reassuring that her health and well-being are more important to them than examination results.

She may need more mothering. Her mother can spend more time talking to her and doing things with her. It is important to listen to her properly, bearing in mind that she is unlikely to be the most demanding or noisiest member of the family. She may need encouraging to pursue any interests and hobbies, especially if they are creative.

If she continues to avoid or refuse food in spite of regular family meals and is avoiding her family and friends, losing weight, and exercising frenetically some other action should be considered.

Onlookers assume that taking a firm stand at the beginning would stop the illness worsening. Unfortunately most parents are unable to tell it is starting. Some parents have stopped anorexia nervosa by applying constant pressure to eat. This is most likely to work either with very young girls or when it coincides with the run-up to examinations or some other hurdle, holding a girl together until this is over. It is better for a father to attempt to do this than the mother.

The father's and the daughter's own anger may combine to give a girl strength and provide a useful diversion from the obstacle she is facing. Once the examinations are taken, the dieting usually stops. The reassurance of her father's concern, combined with the reaffirmation of his paternal role

164

may make her feel more secure, particularly if he is usually too busy to concern himself with his children.

Some mothers claim they have reversed the anorexia nervosa in its early stages by prolonged hysterics. A mother who noticed her daughter's emaciation for the first time on a beach in Kenya said, 'I screamed, yelled and had hysterics for two days without stopping. Everyone in the hotel could hear, I didn't care. My husband was furious, appalled by my behaviour, my other children were humiliated and embarrassed. In the end she started to eat and although she continued to be obsessed with her figure and her diet she put on enough weight to look reasonable and never got any worse.' The Devil or the deep blue sea?

It is well worth trying a short sharp attack, provided it really is short and the mother is strong enough to carry it out without being affected by other people's reactions. The great difficulty is that a mother's first reaction is a paralysing mixture of fear, anger and compassion. She feels prolonged anger would be pointless and unkind.

Quick decisive action may be effective with some girls. Unfortunately a prolonged battering may develop fear, and concern turn into impotent rage. Continuous bullying by a mother is not likely to succeed. Nor are sarcasm, teasing and unkind jokes. A girl may be pushed out of anorexia nervosa in its early stages. She is most unlikely to be laughed out of it.

The more control an anorectic has over her eating, the greater the danger of weight loss. The lower her weight drops the more intense and long lasting are the psychological ill-effects of starvation, altering both her perception and her behaviour until it becomes increasingly difficult to reverse the anorexia nervosa with or without professional help. A daughter who sees her normally calm mother succumbing to paroxysms of impotent rage will feel she is winning. The element of a duel intensifies. The daughter who sees her weight control as her only weapon becomes increasingly and self-destructively reliant upon it.

Attacking potential anorexia nervosa at its beginning may be effective, but it begs the question of why a neurosis such as anorexia nervosa is necessary. Will a rapid reversal merely drive the problems which led to compulsive dieting further into a sufferer, festering until they re-emerge in the same or a different form when she is older.

Is the increase in adolescent neurosis partly due to the modern *laissez-faire* attitude towards bringing up children, allowing an earlier eruption of psychological problems. Are the anorectics of today replacing the depressed middle-aged women of previous generations? It appears that anorexia nervosa which has been controlled during adolescence may manifest later unless the problems which led to it have been resolved.

If extra care combined with a short sharp attack on the dieting have no effect, the parents must obtain a diagnosis. Parents find it hard to understand that it is the lack of self-confidence, the paralysing sense of ineffectiveness under-lying anorexia nervosa, which make it difficult for a girl to relinquish her control. They naturally find it increasingly hard to maintain the strict discipline and routine their daughter needs.

The diagnosis may be made by the family doctor. This may be the first hurdle. Amenorrhoea of at least three months' duration is necessary for a diagnosis of anorexia nervosa. Some girls have never had a period. Some girls' periods have stopped for a year or more before dieting commences, but many girls start compulsive, often secret, dieting well before they cease to menstruate. Thus, if action were taken in the sub-clinical stage, as soon as the weight loss and dieting were noticed, many girls might be saved.

It is no good a doctor telling a mother she is fussing unnecessarily – ignore the problem and it will go away. Anorexia nervosa does not go away. It merely gets worse. Even if a doctor thinks he has a neurotic, over-anxious mother to deal with, it would be sensible, humane and cost-effective to try to cure potential cases of anorexia nervosa at the beginning.

The GP could regularly weigh a girl who is losing weight and consistently refusing to eat or vomiting her food. He could give her a diet sheet and send or give a duplicate one to her mother. The mother will have guidelines for meals with which her daughter cannot reasonably argue. If she continues to refuse food, her doctor and her family will be alerted to the possibility of serious problems, making both action and acceptance easier. The doctor can establish a supportive relationship with her, enabling her to bring up any subjects which may be worrying her. This need take only 10 minutes each week, possibly saving a great deal of time in the long run. It may be a mistake to wait until amenorrhoea has lasted for several months, as by this time severe weight loss can have occurred.

If the weight loss continues, slowly or dramatically, a visit to a consultant psychiatrist could be arranged. A mother can ask to be referred to a consultant if the GP is unwilling to diagnose anorexia nervosa. The doctor may suggest it if he feels unable to deal with a case of anorexia nervosa and has found that specialised help is the best.

A girl may find it a great relief to talk to someone who understands how terrible her obsession with food is for her. She may be dominated by hunger and her need to fight it, feeling that starvation is her key to survival. She may be helped by talking to a doctor who does not treat her as a naughty, silly, little girl. If only doctors would take the time and trouble to explain to parents how their daughter feels and what they can do to help.

It may help a girl and her parents to realise what trouble she is in. Many girls are upset by feelings of deep loathing for one or more members of their family, of acute depression, of running away from growing up. They may need to consider that family tensions or undue educational pressure underlie their dieting. A girl has an opportunity to raise any problems which may worry her, and she may then be able to discuss them with her parents.

Some children are loth to worry their parents with their own troubles when the parents have other difficulties, are too busy, or cannot understand how small worries can magnify. An interview with a psychiatrist which facilitates a family discussion can sometimes reverse the anorexia nervosa, depending how much mutual love and trust exist within the family.

Many people are ashamed of seeing a psychiatrist. It is unkind of parents to boast about it, as though it marks them as being in some way special, or to allow their embarrassment to lead them into making unkind and derogatory remarks.

If the condition worsens it may be easier to be admitted to hospital quickly if a consultant has already been seen. Unless a girl is very ill or wants to go into hospital she will probably be looked after at home. There are some fairly mild cases which respond well to early hospital admission, although the limited medical facilities make this increasingly unlikely.

What can the mother do once she has a diagnosis of anorexia nervosa? She can regard the illness as a medical problem outside her maternal expertise, with the family doctor monitoring her daughter's eating and arranging for in-patient treatment if it becomes necessary. She may be able to arrange for her daughter to be seen regularly by a psychiatrist who is used to dealing with anorexia nervosa. She can ask her family doctor to arrange for her daughter to attend the local hospital as an out-patient. An increasing number of anorectics are treated as out-patients.

The advantage of seeing a psychiatrist privately, bearing in mind that many people have private health insurance which covers the costs, is that parents will have easier access to the doctor and their daughter will always see the same person. It may also mean that she has to take less time off from her studies, as school or college curricula are not geared to out-patient clinics.

The mother may feel that this is her problem and want to look after her daughter herself. She may experience considerable doubts about her ability to help her daughter through anorexia nervosa. She may feel that determined efforts will produce good results but be uncertain whether she has the physical or emotional strength to engage in what may prove to be a long campaign. She may feel it is wrong for a vulnerable girl to be at the receiving end of her mother's determination, spiced with anger and resentment, to force her to eat and put on weight.

She may feel that she will mentally damage her fragile daughter by prolonged pressure, so that in winning the fight she may lose the battle to give her daughter the self-confidence and autonomy which are fundamental to recovery. She may be right. How is she to know?

She cannot know. She can only face reality. Even if she decides that it would be better for her daughter to be looked after by the medical profession the girl will still be living at home most of the time. Hospitals will keep her daughter in only until they feel that she has achieved the adequate stabilised weight which enables her to think rationally, to be out of physical danger and to have reached a state from which further recovery is possible. This may not work. Many girls are readmitted to hospital several times before they are able to continue their development with a sustained recovery. Both the renewed weight loss prior to readmission and the hospital visiting involve the mother in additional strain.

Therefore, whether she likes it or not, the mother will probably have to provide a base for her daughter, ensuring she is properly cared for while not being allowed to disrupt the family by causing ungovernable chaos.

The mother's first task is to restore her daughter's weight. The weight loss must be stopped and reversed as soon as possible. It may be a year or more before the weight reaches an acceptable target.

The mother may accept that anorexia nervosa has to run

its natural course, during which she must continue to try to persuade her daughter to eat normally and with other people. She may see her role as mounting a 'holding operation', making sure that her daughter maintains enough weight to be able to function normally, hoping that one day either a miracle, a boy friend or the natural course of events will cure the anorexia nervosa.

She realises she may have to alter course if her daughter becomes much iller or if the strain on any other member or members of the family becomes too great. The mother needs to create a strong, supportive structure, while at the same time remaining alert for the need to change tactics, reminding herself constantly that she must think of improvement in terms of months or even years, rather than of weeks or days.

If the weight loss is allowed to continue unchecked her daughter will be in increasing physical and psychological danger. Anorectics die from inanition – having no calories left. They die, after many years, from suicide born of their despair and depression. Their bodies eventually start feeding on the protein in the muscles. When the heart muscle weakens it can lead to irregularities in rhythms and even congestive heart failure. Both anorexia nervosa and bulimia nervosa can destroy the body's delicate balance of electrolytes, particularly potassium, so causing serious cardiac abnormalities.

Continual underweight can lead to insomnia, depersonalisation, depression, irritability and lack of concentration. All of these make it more difficult for an anorectic to be helped or to help herself.

The mother of a daughter with anorexia nervosa has to use her head, and keep her heart firmly under control. Both she and her daughter need to switch from emotional to cerebral functioning. The mother has to abandon any notions she may harbour about being the 'good' parent. Fathers frequently refer to the wife as the 'caring' parent, bearing the problems and burdens. The mother has to care enough about her daughter not to mind if she and everyone else in the family seem to hate her, doing everything they can to frustrate her efforts.

Anorexia nervosa is a cry for help. A girl's own expectations and those of others may have combined to overwhelm her. She is undergoing an intense adolescent identity crisis, trying to establish who or what she is before feeling strong enough to continue to the next stage of her development. She needs reassurance, firmness and an absolute refusal to allow any 'games' to develop. She needs to know that her entire family are united in their efforts to help her out of what she does not see as an illness. Advice given to parents of anorectics inevitably sounds hard and even vindictive because the illness is not properly explained to them.

The daughter needs time spending on her and with her to help her feel less worthless and insignificant. Parents are not always aware how totally defeated a girl may be by a dominant sibling, either older or younger. Since the strong have no need to be devious the parents may find the dominant child in their family is the most straightforward and easiest with whom to communicate.

The strength of an anorectic has always seemed to me to be grossly over-rated and misunderstood. The strength of will is a measure of the depth of her despair, illustrating the difficulties she has in surviving, rather than evidence of a will of megalomaniac proportions. 'She must be strong to have anorexia nervosa' betrays misunderstanding of the strength of the instinct to survive. This may have been lost sight of in societies where survival is expected. An anorectic may resemble her mother in that her constitutional strength belies her difficulties in asserting herself.

Parents of an anorectic daughter are frightened and confused by the apparent change of personality which prolonged starvation can produce. They do not realise their daughter's underlying personality is the same. Once she is better she will be the same girl they know and love. She will no longer, however, be a little girl who relies totally upon her parents, accepting their views and behaviour as automatically right. She will be older, more adult and tempered by an unhappy and destructive experience.

Parents must never despair but neither should they hope for too much too soon. A mother found T. S. Eliot's words helpful:

> I said to my soul, be still, and wait without hope
> For hope would be hope for the wrong thing . . .
> East Coker', III

Even severe cases of several years' duration can be reversed rapidly, as I know from personal experience. This may involve two factors. The willingness of the mother, combined with her own need to survive, to rise above the illness and establish control. This may unconsciously coincide with her daughter experiencing the moment of 'being at the bottom of the pit' which is often the turning point in self-destruction.

It is essential to be well organised. Shopping planned around a weekly menu helps to allay the anxiety over shopping and cooking which are part of a mother's early and continuing reaction to anorexia nervosa. It also helps her to keep a check on her housekeeping money.

The anorectic's dishonesty over her intake of food extends to a ruthless determination to buy and eat whatever she wants. This may include large quantities of laxatives. She cannot help herself. It does not mean that dishonesty is an ineradicable part of a sadly altered personality. Her basic personality will return to view once she has conquered and been helped to conquer her obsession with food and her view of emaciation as triumph.

Once the loss of weight which leads to her disorganised thinking has been reversed, she will be able to accept that triumph is only the other side of failure and that failure in one area does not mean annihilation in all others. The fear of being fat, said with many girls to be greater than the fear of death, has to be less than the fear of constant attention and lack of freedom which a relentlessly determined mother may come to represent.

The mother has to decide how to tackle the food problem. This can rapidly become chaotic, so the sooner a rigid routine is imposed upon family eating the better it will be. She may find it helpful to return to the routine she had when her children were small.

She needs to be present at every meal including breakfast. Normally, anorectics are honest and reliable but they are completely untrustworthy where food is concerned. No mother can believe her daughter's account of what she has eaten at a meal unless she has actually seen her eating and swallowing it. She must then prevent her daughter getting to a lavatory for at least one hour. Some mothers lock the lavatory doors before a meal begins so that their daughters cannot nip in to be sick after it.

The mother must control her cooking, shopping and kitchen. It is a mistake to do food shopping with an anorectic daughter, allowing her to choose her own food in the hope that she will eat it. She should not allow her daughter to cook since the most effective way of stopping an incipient obsession with food is to prevent it starting. A mother whose daughter is already obsessed with food and trying to take over the kitchen must make determined efforts to stop her doing so. Some mothers find it helpful to keep the kitchen and larder locked unless they are in there themselves.

The mother must not allow herself to be bamboozled into buying extra recipe books or magazines about food. Her daughter's interest in cooking is not a good sign but a continuing symptom. Her daughter needs distracting from food. Anorexia nervosa occurs in families who are professionally involved with food. Their livelihood has become the girl's obsession. Cookery schools are more aware of the dangers of the anorectic's obsession with food and some refuse to take anorectics or ex-anorectics as students.

173

There may be an argument for applying the psychiatric technique of 'flooding' to an anorectic, surrounding her with food, recipes, photographs of food, spending hours every day cooking with her until she can bear it no longer. Were I starting again I would probably try this if no results were being obtained from more orthodox methods.

A mother whose daughter binges has to do her best to make it impossible for her. If she finds food vanishing from the larder, refrigerator and freezer she may find it helpful to make a list of every item of food, pinning it to the wall and asking her family to tick off anything they have eaten. If her daughter is hiding food under her bed, in cupboards, behind the bookshelves, her mother can take out everything she can find each morning, leaving it conspicuously in the middle of the room. Her daughter may be very relieved to be caught. It is most important never to turn a blind eye to any unusual behaviour with food.

What can a mother do if her daughter completely refuses to eat, retiring to her bedroom and locking the door as a meal approaches. First, take away the key. Second, experience has shown that if a mother spends time with her daughter, remaining with her firmly but as calmly as possible she may eventually come into the kitchen or dining room. She may find it necessary to dog her daughter's footsteps until the poor girl realises that the anorexia nervosa is producing more control over her than she had to endure without it, obtaining exactly the opposite result to the one she unconsciously intended. A continual refusal to eat is her way of establishing control over her mother, so her mother must not make any allowances for the anorexia nervosa. If she misses a meal her mother must not cook for her at another time or allow her to help herself.

The mother should try not to resort to subterfuge. She must not leave food lying around in the hope that her daughter will help herself when no one is looking. This again avoids the central issue. It is neither kind nor caring to be other than firm about the family eating. The greatest help a mother can give her daughter is to make it impossible for her to control it. It can seem ungrateful to forbid a daughter to cook for the family, usually rich, delicious food, which she will enjoy watching everyone except herself swallowing. In allowing her to do so a mother is relinquishing her maternal role, both allowing her daughter to assume and imposing upon her an inappropriate responsibility.

Previous generations of children never ate alone. The inevitable consequence of the increase in convenience and junk food and of so many women working is that it has become easy for mothers to tell their children to help themselves or to take something from the freezer. Sloppy eating habits and families who no longer regularly eat together may also be signs of underlying tensions and family troubles.

A mother may attempt to refeed her daughter by lovingly and patiently coaxing her to eat every mouthful for months on end. This usually only works if mother and daughter can be alone for meals.

A desperately worried mother may make the mistake of allowing an adolescent daughter to resume the role of a baby, sitting on her lap to be spoon-fed. A girl must continue to behave, and her family behave towards her, as though she were well. The mother must not start or encourage a babying process by making sure her daughter sits beside her at every meal. The girl needs to be integrated with the rest of the family. Extra time and attention given to her at mealtimes damages her relationship with her siblings. They are usually unable to resist joining in the fray, taking and frequently changing sides, while regarding her as a nuisance whose behaviour is beyond normal comprehension.

No meal should be allowed to drag on for too long. If a girl takes more than ten minutes longer than any of the rest of the family to finish her food the mother should throw away her daughter's meal. Once she starts to make special allowances she is sunk. The downward spiral of emotional blackmail is set in motion, making the duration and process of the illness long and difficult.

A mother may be uncertain about the amount of weight her daughter should put on each week. When my daughter was determined to get better we made a plan together. We set a deadline of eight weeks, in the first seven of which she was to gain 9.5kg (21lb) keeping it steady for the last week before we went on holiday. She tried to gain 1.5kg (3lb) in the first two days of each week so that she then had five days to keep the weight gain steady and to adjust to it. This worked reasonably well although the first few weeks were difficult for her and she had bouts of panic and anger. As her weight increased so did her confidence and her determination to succeed. And so did mine.

It is unfair to expect a daughter to eat vegetables swimming in butter or rich puddings. Mothers of anorectics sometimes mention the weight they themselves have put on during the anorexia nervosa. 'Look what it's done to me,' they wail despondently. This is partly a result of the general dietary chaos. Perversity, panic or excessive zeal may lead a mother to cook more and richer food than before. The daughter's refusal to eat the results of her efforts increases her mother's anger. This in turn makes the siblings even more angry. The anorectic daughter feels increasingly helpless, permanently in the wrong. It is even more necessary for her to establish herself as her own person – dieting seems to her the only way to do this.

A mother who has been depressed for a long time may unwittingly contribute to her daughter's condition by allowing her to take over the cooking while the mother becomes apathetic and emotionally absent from her family. She may have been ill herself, absorbed by the needs of older relations or by a job and so grateful for her teenage daughter's help. The poor girl may have felt that this was the only way she was likely to be fed.

A mother who feels guilty about this may see her daughter's help as an attempt at domination. It may take a long time for a mother to reassume control of her most usual function – cooking for her family. Anorexia nervosa undermines a mother at the most basic level. A mother who feels that she has failed can be easily manoeuvred from her normal control of her kitchen.

A mother may become so involved in what is going on that she is unable to realise that her daughter's control is being allowed to grow. She may not know when or how she is being controlled.

She is being controlled when she allows her daughter to do her own cooking when she wants, giving into her demands to be allowed to use the kitchen which she often leaves in a mess. She is being controlled when she buys special food for her daughter or allows her to buy her own.

She is being controlled when she stops the siblings doing things they would normally do because they might upset or undermine their sister, making her feel left out and isolated.

She is being controlled when she feels guilty about leaving the house without her daughter's permission, or when she feels she ought to be in the house when her daughter comes home.

She is being controlled when she is aware day and night of every move her daughter makes, failing to make a stand about behaviour she would not tolerate from anyone else – being woken by the sound of hectic exercising at 4 a.m. or nauseated by the disgusting smell of stale overcooked cabbage at all hours of the day and night.

She is being controlled when she is afraid that anything and everything she does might upset her daughter. Or when she is hypersensitive to the effect anyone else might have on her daughter, failing to realise that she may also be upsetting them. She is being controlled when she allows her daughter to telephone her a dozen or more times a day and does not leave the telephone off the hook.

She is being controlled whenever she turns a blind eye to her daughter's anti-social behaviour and when she is always making excuses for her, particularly about her non-attendance at school, college or job.

She is being controlled when she is habitually kicked or has her hair pulled by her daughter and does not turn round and slap her. She is being controlled when she is afraid to leave the room.

She can keep in touch with reality by repeating to herself 'What would I do if she did not have anorexia nervosa?' and then doing it.

A mother may be confused by the apparently conflicting advice she is given. She may not understand why she must exert additional control over a daughter who is partly ill because she feels over-controlled. The problem is one of boundaries. These may have been weak before the anorexia nervosa developed and by the time help is sought may have disintegrated altogether in the general chaos. The mother needs to control everything which comes into her domestic province. She does not need to control her daughter's thoughts, friends, homework, sex life, ambitions, expectations, political opinions, or choice of clothes, provided she is not expected to pay for them.

A mother must retain control over her own money. She can help her daughter by making it difficult if not impossible for her to go on spending sprees. The terror of the shoplifting to which some anorectics are prone unfortunately leads unwary parents into slackness about money. There is obviously no need to treat a girl as irresponsible by altering or removing her regular pocket money or allowance. If a girl who is working is spending all her money on food her parents must not be tempted to give her extra money for clothes, entertainment or anything else. She needs to be responsible for herself.

Doctors insist that shoplifting is not the worst thing that can happen when a girl is anorectic. Mothers are horrified by a point of view which convinces them that most psychiatrists are mad. It is hard to realise that it may only be by getting into trouble that a girl can understand fully what trouble she is in.

The more her mother panders to her little whims the more difficult she makes it for her daughter to be adult in her behaviour. The thinner and iller her daughter becomes, the more concerned the mother becomes, the more she searches for a way to restore her daughter's hopes and therefore health; the more the mother gives into her daughter's demands, the greater do the peripheral benefits of anorexia nervosa seem, and the less likely is her daughter to see any advantage in being well again.

As the illness continues and begins to affect the family structure, increasing the mother's worry, the more any change can seem like an improvement. It is at this stage that collusion centring on food and money may be easily and unconsciously established. The mother, hoping a little treat may make her daughter more agreeable and more prepared to eat, begins to ask what she would like to eat and to do. This is often the first bad mistake. Allowing her gradually to assume that she is entitled to behave differently from other people will very soon make her feel that she will only continue to receive attention (equated in her mind with love) for as long as she continues to be different.

While anorexia nervosa must not be ignored, neither should it be allowed to dominate a family. It is a depressive illness and depression is depressing. It is entirely negative and made worse by the sufferer's genuine inability to see that she is ill. She resists help partly because she can see no need for it and often cannot understand why people think she needs to get better. She is in a state of constant fear. She is afraid of the storms and anger that she arouses, afraid of going to hospital, afraid of death, afraid of worse disintegration of an increasingly shaky family structure, afraid of what will happen to her if she does get 'better', afraid of losing control, afraid of maintaining it, but above all, quite outweighing her other fears, she is afraid of being fat. Fat, moreover, by her new standards rather than by those of other people.

Prolonged stress and a sense of proportion are not compatible. Many mothers remember a time when the whole family seemed to be engulfed in a kind of madness. For this the mother may largely be to blame. She felt at the time a helpless failure, afterwards she sees that she was foolish and ignorant. She was unable to deal rationally with even the simplest problems. There was constant conflict and dissension within the family, accusations flying around, even the smallest mishap being regarded with fear and suspicion.

Mothers recall how they blamed their anorectic daughter for everything that went wrong. They blamed her for their own inability to cope, they blamed her for the way in which hidden tensions came to the surface, they blamed her for the way in which they lost contact with friends, for spoiling their summer holidays, for developing a condition which brought their own shortcomings to light, they blamed her for any deterioration in her siblings' behaviour. The mothers thought they were blaming anorexia nervosa. She felt that they were blaming her.

The position of a girl with anorexia nervosa within her own family is initially difficult and can swiftly become completely impossible. She is neither old enough nor mature enough to stand firm against the emotional onslaughts to which she may be subjected. She is as bewildered by everyone's reaction to the anorexia nervosa as they are by its existence. She can see nothing wrong with her emaciation and obsession with food and so can see no point in getting better.

As the illness progresses and her daughter becomes more

'child-like' a mother finds it increasingly difficult to see the point of pretending that she is, or nearly is, an adult. This may be more difficult with a young adolescent than it is with an older girl whose anorexia nervosa may have developed as the result of an unhappy sexual experience.

While a mother may find it easier to help a young (primary) anorectic as she is still young enough to be expected to do what she is told, and to accept some authority from her parents, school or doctor, there is a much longer time until she can reasonably be expected to detach emotionally if not physically from her mother. If the condition shows no real sign of improvement within a fairly short time, say up to one year, the mother is going to have to sit it out. She has to accept that it may last for several years, during which there are bound to be ups and downs and disappointments. Until her daughter is old enough to begin to live her own life she has no alternative to doing her best and allowing the illness to cause as little disruption as possible.

There is a great deal of anger in anorexia nervosa. Both the sufferer and everyone else feel extremely angry far too often. The anger needs to be dispersed, as anorexia nervosa is an illness which festers like a boil. Like a boil, it has to burst and the poison allowed to drain away before a healing process can begin. It is no good being afraid or backing down in front of other people.

Some of the methods used by psychiatrists which are so unacceptable to parents are directed to releasing the rage which eats into a girl, blocking her recovery. The terrible frustration contained in anorexia nervosa has to have an outlet. A daughter may look frail and is obviously suffering intensely. She is not too frail to release her tension by being allowed or made to be angry. Like many other mothers, I can remember the times when my daughter's anger boiled in her so hard that I allowed myself to evade issues, to accept insult, to exhibit each and every sign of moral cowardice rather than risk an explosion.

181

A mother may feel that she would be able to do more to help her daughter if she only knew what she was feeling or thinking. It is hard to know what a girl with anorexia nervosa really feels – most girls reel off a standard description of what they say they have been told they feel. Many are unsure how much of this they believe.

My daughter told me recently that having anorexia nervosa was like being in a coma for four years. She was far less aware of us than we were of her. We came increasingly, I think, to have only a nuisance value. We hovered on the edge of her consciousness. We made forays into her haze and had to be banished. We disturbed her concentration on food and her anorectic world. Other girls told me that neither observation nor neglect seemed to help them.

The parallel with a coma is apt. Sometimes contact can be made. There are long periods of waiting. There are moments of great joy when the patient seems to be pulling herself back into contact with her family, when a short conversation can seem like a door opening into a new and better world. There are the bad moments, too, when your daughter flinches from you, refusing to touch anything you have touched.

Patience and understanding are necessary. Both are open to interpretation. Patience has largely passive connotations but should imply continuing tolerance with what cannot at the moment be altered rather than general inertia. Activity, distraction, noise, unpredictability of action (but not of response and constant support, faith and love), talk, fun are needed. She needs to be involved in what goes on around her, dragged out for walks, kept occupied, braced up, doing things with her family even when she is rejecting them. A mother needs the patience not to give up, to keep going, to refuse to allow herself to be driven mad or obsessed by the anorexia nervosa.

Various kinds of understanding are needed. The mother has to understand the effect her daughter's obsession with food is having on her. She must understand that understanding has limits and must not allow bloody-minded behaviour, under the delusion – or because she cannot be bothered to argue – that this is the best way for her daughter to find herself. She must understand that her daughter needs boundaries and will feel more secure once she knows what these are. She must understand that the illness is placing a great strain on her husband and children, as well as on her extended family and friends. She must understand that they cannot understand why she is making quite such heavy weather of it. No one who has not experienced it can understand the demoralising effect and constant heartache of living with a child in a state of chronic suicide. She must understand that she may be confusing anorectic behaviour with difficult teenage behaviour and so exaggerating the difficulties.

A mother understands that if she is to help her daughter to regain self-confidence and self-respect, without which she cannot recover, she has to find a way to detach emotionally, sometimes physically, from her without leaving a legacy of bitterness and hurt. She may find it hard to detach because she has adjusted to her new role and fears further upheaval. She may feel it is irresponsible not to spend all her time with her daughter. An anorectic needs to feel that her mother is on her side rather than at her side. She needs her mother to be firmly behind her so that she cannot take a step backwards rather than to actually push her forwards.

A girl suffering from anorexia nervosa will develop increasing self-confidence when she feels able to act on her own initiative, withstanding any failures without resorting again to anorexia nervosa. Her self-respect develops with her self-confidence, making it easier for her to respect and accept other people.

A mother can help her daughter to regain her self-respect by respecting her for herself. She has to treat her as she would any other girl or young adult of her age. This may be difficult.

A mother whose daughter first developed anorexia nervosa in her early teens may continue to behave towards her as though she has never grown any older. The longer the illness lasts the more difficult she finds it to adjust to her daughter's chronological age, especially as even recovered anorectics look much younger than they really are. If a mother can spend time with friends whose daughters are the same age and encourage her own daughter to see friends she may find this easier.

An anorectic girl may lose all contact with her friends and peers unless she is genuinely encouraged to see them. The withdrawal from friends and family is as painful to watch as it must be to endure. The only help a mother can give her daughter is to encourage her to keep in contact with them. A daughter has to re-establish relationships and form new friendships herself. This may involve whispered telephone conversations, hidden letters, meeting away from home and so on. Many anorectics say that their mothers have a habit of comparing them with other girls and saying, 'Thank goodness you're not like that', or always referring to their friends as 'little'. This forces them to be different from their contemporaries at an age when conformity may be essential. Some girls are embarrassed by their mothers' efforts to please them, fussing over them and their friends so that they feel helpless and frustrated.

A mother has considerable difficulty in helping the daughter to maintain contact with her contemporaries. She will isolate herself rather than conform to their way of life, this isolation naturally making her more depressed. There is the added problem that her friends' mothers may understandably discourage their own daughters' friendship with her because they do not wish them to develop anorexia nervosa.

As a girl begins to recover she will find it much easier to enjoy being with other people, and with reasonable luck and a certain amount of effort the situation should reverse itself. Her mother will have to help to get her going again by being prepared to entertain anyone and everyone at short notice and as often as possible. No opportunity should be missed to widen her daughter's circle of friends and activities.

A mother who sees plenty of other adolescents may find it easier to understand how things have changed since she was young. Mothers of daughters with anorexia nervosa range in age from the mid-30s to the late 70s, covering several generations. For most, the change in attitude and behaviour of adolescents during the last 15 or 20 years appears to be a symbol of the decadence to which we have unwittingly contributed. We did not necessarily avoid self-destructive behaviour because we were better brought up, had instilled in us earlier better moral principles or were more fundamentally stable, but we differed from the present generation in that we were not subjected to the pressures of modern youth and did not have so many options available to us.

We were not expected to perform, we were not subjected to the pressure of modern advertising. Make-up, fashionable clothes, alcohol, cigarettes, hard and soft drugs and contraceptives were not available to us. We were not as politically or socially aware as children are now and we did not have our lessons infiltrated with left-wing ideals, some of which appear to have been designed to encourage children to reject their parents' standards and values. We did not have sexual education either at such an early age or in such detail as children do now. We were controlled to some extent by fear – fear of our parents, especially our fathers, fear of God, fear of disgrace, fear of pregnancy. Fear is now unacceptable but when one looks at the enormous increase in the level of anxiety to which its absence may have largely contributed, it no longer seems so bad.

Clothes are often a problem. As a girl becomes increasingly emaciated and withdrawn her appearance may deteriorate. She may begin to wear the same clothes every day, the dirtier and more dilapidated the better. Her appearance attracts attention and her mother begins to feel she is doing it for this reason. She tries to ignore her daughter's appearance, 'Just another phase she is going through', defending her against criticism while unable to resist criticising her herself. She feels she must do everything she can to improve her daughter's appearance and so restore her self-respect.

New clothes are bought – often costing more than parents can afford and laying the daughter open once again to charges of being a spoilt child – in the hope that by looking better she will feel better. The new clothes are seldom worn. After the initial enthusiasm they may be put away in a cupboard, never to be seen again. The siblings are furious, the anorectic continues to wear her grubby jeans, the parents fulminate and despair.

A mother who is saddened to see her daughter looking like a neglected waif and stray has to harden her heart, ignoring it as much as she can. If she panders to her daughter's demands for clothes she will enable her to continue and increase her control over her family. She may want to encourage her daughter by telling her how nice she looks but must remember the cardinal rule that never under any circumstances should she or anyone else refer to her daughter's physical appearance. 'You do look pretty and/or well' is translated by an anorectic as meaning that she has put on weight and must lose it again as soon as possible. 'You look ill/too thin/scrawny/like something out of Belsen' means to her that she must be losing weight noticeably and that if she continues to diet so successfully will soon be even thinner.

A girl with anorexia nervosa will take more interest in her appearance as her weight and self-confidence improve. She needs to be encouraged to choose her own clothes; some girls like to make them for themselves. Some mothers use clothes as an incentive, buying something really pretty that will fit a girl once she has achieved a normal weight.

Many anorectics feel that they are chronic failures. The sense of failure may have started when they were young, often without the parents being aware of it. Failure to get into the school she or her parents wanted her to go to or being taken away from a boarding school at which she was unhappy may have started it. Parents may feel guilty about making the original decision about her education and so try to compensate by allowing her to escape from other awkward situations. It is difficult for a girl to stick to anything once she is in the habit of failing and of giving up.

Having started a course or job she must, for her own good, either finish it or stick at it for at least three months. Every time she gives up anything she finds difficult she takes a step backwards. If she tends to be depressed she needs to be occupied as much as possible, so parents must not worry too much if they find it necessary to be tougher with her than they would like to be. If she is having problems at work she must be allowed to sort them out for herself even though her mother may feel she is not able to protect herself properly. She needs outlets into which to channel her tremendous determination and perseverance.

There is the question of the comparative value to an anorectic of qualifications and experience. Parents of any vulnerable child tend to emphasise the child's extra need for qualifications. This may mean a girl is stretched too hard and too fast. It may mean she is delaying the time when she can be independent. It is hard for parents to know what to do. Unless an anorectic has a burning ambition or particular talent it is probably best for her to be self-supporting as soon as possible.

Parents may have difficulty in coming to terms with the end of their hopes, especially when her education has meant years of financial strain. They may be bitter and embarrassed when their daughter takes a job which does not meet their expectations. They must encourage her to make her own decisions even if some of them are unexpected or unwelcome. 'This is the first positive thing I've done' is how a daughter feels when she resists her parents' ambitions or expectations. She needs to function in her own way and at her own speed without their financial support. A girl who is living at home will feel better if she contributes something to the housekeeping.

It is harder for a mother whose daughter is still at school to help her build up her self-confidence. Mothers often try to give daughters some special responsibility. They can enlist their daughters' help in different ways without feeling inadequate themselves. No woman needs to be hyper-efficient and competent all the time. Anorectics say, 'My mother is so good at everything I feel I can never live up to her.'

Anyone who has been as ill and as difficult to live with as an anorectic has a real need to be able to give. It is hurtful and humiliating to be always at the receiving end, always saying thank you, always bearing the burden of continual gratitude. It may be more blessed to give than to receive but it is also more pleasant and much easier.

A mother may be upset by the large number of Christmas presents her daughter often gives her, feeling guilty and ashamed. She may over-react emotionally – why can't she eat a normal meal instead? She feels confused, her thanks seem inadequate – her daughter feels like this all the rest of the year.

Christmas is always a difficult time for anorectics and their families. The extra food induces extra rage. Parents may not realise how much their daughter is longing to eat, the extra food meaning she has to summon up additional will to refuse it. A girl who binges may be unable to resist devouring an enormous and possibly dangerous amount of food. She may use her inability to control her appetite as an excuse not to come home for Christmas. Friends can help by asking the family to have meals with them over Christmas, provided they are not going to be infuriated by her refusal to eat everything they produce.

A mother is embarrassed and a hostess irritated by trying to feed a girl, however pretty she may be, who is not

188

prepared or able to make an effort to be agreeable, and who apparently has no compunction whatever about spoiling other people's fun. A girl may be too frightened of being forced to eat to be able to join in. Once she has recovered, her social problems will probably disappear.

How is a mother to know when her daughter is cured? How is recovery assessed? A girl is cured when her weight has been restored, when she eats with her family or other people, when she is neither eating nor bingeing secretly, when she has stopped vomiting; when she shows no signs of abnormal or obsessive behaviour, when her attitudes are more or less the same as those of any other girl of her age and education, even if these are not acceptable to her parents; when menstruation is resumed.

A mother may find it helpful to see recovery as a pro-longed convalescence, starting when weight has been re-gained and stabilised and leading hopefully to a cure. This may take a year or more.

A girl needs to hold her target weight with only slight variations for at least one year. Even after this there may be relapses. A sudden increase in weight may indicate that she is bingeing. She is not better if she is controlling her weight by vomiting or laxative abuse, if she eats alone, or if she compulsively over-eats. She may continue to be faddy about food, like a great many people who are not anorectic, but she should be able to eat at least something of what other people are eating at meals.

She needs gradually to become more socially aggressive. Many girls find social occasions difficult to face but this should improve with time and encouragement. The longer a girl has been isolated the more difficult she finds it to reintegrate with her contemporaries. As she gets better she may bitterly regret the wasted years, feeling hopelessly out of step with her friends. She feels a failure when she hears them talking about all the things they may have been doing while she has been ill. She has nothing to tell. A mother may accept that her daughter finds safety in isolation for a time, but she herself continues to see her own friends as much as possible. The isolation may embrace the whole family so that any of their activities may indirectly help the daughter.

She may make friends while she is in hospital. She may be helped by joining a self-help group, as the exchange of views and experiences may make her feel less lonely and less peculiar. She may feel better once she realises how many other girls are in her situation, understanding her feelings of inadequacy and insecurity better than outsiders to whom anorectics seem both capable and cared for. Mothers who have been to self-help meetings have sometimes been alarmed by seeing girls who have been anorectic for many years, but have generally found that they have been able to discuss anorexia nervosa more rationally with their daughters afterwards.

The great problem for self-help groups, of which they are well aware, is that they concentrate people's attention on one problem. Members enjoy, especially if they have been isolated for some time, having the opportunity of meeting other parents or sufferers and of making new friends. There is a danger of meetings and contacts becoming increasingly valued for their social content and so lessening the wish for recovery. The principle of supply and demand may mean that the setting up of a system to deal with a specific problem may ensure its continuation and even encourage it.

Anorectics need, like all adolescents, to widen their circle of friends and to feel accepted within their peer group. Girls with anorexia nervosa may initially receive a great deal of attention, some of it too intense for them to be able to cope with, but as the illness is an anti-social one this may dwindle away to practically nothing. Their natural shyness may have always made communication difficult and there is some truth in the view that a girl with even one really close friend would be unlikely to drift into anorexia nervosa. A girl may reject the help of her friends because they see forcing food upon her as the best way to help her. The more they try to do this the more she rejects them. The more she rejects them the more unwilling they become to make any effort to help her and the cessation of their attempts increases her feeling of rejection.

Friends who want to help can do so by taking her out with them, talking to her and trying to involve her in what is going on, but without pressing food upon her or commenting on her thinness. A loyal and undemanding friend can do a great deal to help, although when the illness is at its worst friends may indeed wonder why they bother.

A girl with anorexia nervosa is afraid of being 'disloyal', feeling guilty and miserable when she discusses or complains about her parents. She may not realise that this is a normal and indeed necessary stage of adolescent development. She needs to compare her family with those of her friends without feeling that it is wrong to be critical or unhappy. She may not realise that looking at her family objectively will help her to love and understand them. She particularly needs to see her mother objectively and in a more balanced way than she has been able to do.

She needs to meet and talk to as many different people as possible. She needs to exchange ideas both with her friends and with people of different ages. She may find that discussing her parents with her grandparents will enable her to understand them better. She needs to be exposed to different points of view and influences so that she may use her own judgement.

She needs to learn to drive as soon as possible, particularly if public transport is unsatisfactory. Difficulties in getting about make her isolation and dependence worse. It is important for her to do things outside her home as there is a risk of her developing agoraphobia.

A mother's own friends would like to help but do not know what to do. They can help by giving mother and daughter a short break from one another. A mother needs to get away from home regularly and to talk to at least one close friend. Friends may never know how deeply grateful a mother is to them for their many kindnesses and for their willingness to listen patiently as she repeats her worries.

An anorectic is well aware that her mother discusses the anorexia nervosa with her friends, hoping for the informed advice few are able to give. The mother needs to talk about it, and her friends, who have known her daughter for most or all of her life, feel increasingly sorry for her. It is her daughter who needs their sympathy and help; she knows that some of them see her as a very tiresome girl, spoilt and difficult. She needs more than anything to feel accepted, so the subtle rejection by adults whom she has known since infancy is damaging and almost impossible for her to combat. The greatest help a mother's friends can give is to take her anorectic daughter out, but without offering her food, preferably arranging it with her directly rather than discussing it with the mother first.

'My mother never hugged and kissed me.' An anorectic daughter may also find it difficult to show her emotions and feelings. Her isolation makes physical contact increasingly unlikely. A mother whose daughter refuses to be touched by her may find that showing more open affection to other members of the family makes it easier for them to show physical affection. Mothers say that their husbands seldom put an arm round them or kiss them in front of the children. The more demonstrative a family can be the easier the anorectic daughter will find it to accept and tolerate physical contact.

It may not be until she is able to accept physical affection within her own family that a girl can face the prospect of having a boy friend. Most anorectics are frightened of boys and have difficulty communicating with them. Some are terrified of being seduced, others feel guilty about any pleasure which can be seen as self-indulgent, some are emotionally nervous. Some girls may be afraid of their mothers' or siblings' jealousy.

A girl with anorexia nervosa may be able to spend time with friends who have brothers or fathers with whom they get on. It may be good for her to work with men, as admiration without the threat of involvement is good for her morale. If she is naive she may be vulnerable to wolves and/or married men. She may be happiest with a slightly passive boy friend who is kind and patient, as it may take her a long time to lose her fear of being touched. Some girls make a 'transitory' marriage in which they are able to come to terms with their sexuality, then remarry on a more stable basis.

A mother may wonder if and when her daughter should leave home. Some girls prefer not to return home from hospital, others have already left home before the anorexia nervosa begins. A girl whose family come from another country may need to return there if she feels more secure living where she feels she belongs and where her friends are.

When should a mother encourage her daughter to live independently? When her daughter feels ready to do so or when the tensions at home are preventing her developing. If she lives in a flat or room her mother must allow her to look after it herself, as rushing round with the duster or doing her ironing will not enable her daughter to achieve the independence she needs. Social workers or the Citizens' Advice Bureau may be able to advise mothers or their daughters about suitable hostels. Sometimes sheltered accommodation and employment can be found for her until she is well enough to manage alone.

Mothers are worried about their daughters' failure to menstruate. Menstruation may start quite quickly after weight has been restored or it may take years. Mothers find quite often that a girl does not menstruate until she has a boy friend. Artificially-induced menstruation is not recommended, so mothers must try not to fuss too much. Both mother and daughter may be concerned that she will not be able to become pregnant.

The mother also has to recover. She needs to look forward

with hope rather than backward with regret. As the years have passed since the anorexia nervosa developed she should have tried to pick up the threads of her life and widened her interests, perhaps finding a job or working for a degree. It is of the utmost importance to do so because the greatest barrier to her daughter's recovery is her mother's fear that nothing lies ahead and that she will have lost her only role, which though worrying and exhausting was also absorbing.

Parental ill-health after an anorectic daughter has recovered may illustrate their fear and may partly be the result of the stress being released. Both parents need to go on developing their own lives, or difficulties will ensue for other members of their family. The positive aspect of anorexia nervosa is that it can sometimes provide a starting point for other members of an anorectic's family, enabling them to grow and develop so that never again is psychosomatic illness necessary.

SCHOOLS AND COLLEGES

Schools and colleges need information from a girl's doctor or family about her general health, her meals, and how to treat and help her. A mother can ask the doctor to write to the headmistress explaining what the school should do.

It is hard for a school with no experience of anorexia nervosa to understand why a girl who looks emaciated and exhausted should not be allowed to go home or to the sickroom whenever she feels like it. If she is feeling ill it is better for her to be allowed to lie down for an hour and then sent back to her classroom than for her mother or housemistress to be telephoned and asked to collect her. The school will not help her by allowing her to give her homework in late, not to do it at all, or to say she was too tired to attempt it but will try to do it another time. Even a small amount of work badly done is better than nothing. She needs to feel that her school, like her family, are supportive but firm.

The school needs to be clear about her eating arrangements. If she is able to eat school meals then she must do so, even if in small quantities. If she really cannot do this it may be better for her to take a packed lunch which must be eaten under the eye of whoever is supervising lunch. She may try all sorts of excuses to avoid eating – music practice, tummy ache, headache, looking for lost books, feeling sick, all of which should be ignored. If she eats and then vomits her food, she needs to be kept away from the lavatory or cloakroom, where she may have a supply of plastic bags, for at least one hour so that she has digested a reasonable amount of the meal.

The sensible practice is developing in some girls' boarding schools of automatically giving a girl who is obviously losing weight extra milk and biscuits at break, tea time and bedtime until her weight is restored to an acceptable level. This is usually supervised by the school matron or housemistress. Parents should allow the school to try this, as the extra attention and cosseting may be all she needs if she is unhappy, homesick or worried. Mothers can ask the school doctor to write both to them and to their GP explaining any regime or treatment which has been started so that it can be continued during the holidays.

A girl's headmistress or housemistress may be able to give a girl reassurance, but it is neither kind nor sensible to probe too deeply into the possible reasons for her troubles as she may easily resent this, becoming more determined than ever to lose weight. Anorexia nervosa needs to be treated as matter-of-factly as possible.

Unfortunately, in some boarding schools girls are able to isolate themselves, creeping off alone to the dormitory to sit and brood and escape the noise of the common rooms. It is an ideal opportunity to exercise unobserved. The school can help by making sure that a girl cannot isolate herself in this way. They can also help by arranging for a girl whose parents live abroad or are for some reason unavailable to be taken out by a relation or another girl's parents whenever there is a school exeat.

It may be necessary for a girl to leave school if she becomes really ill. She cannot be expected to work when she is seriously ill although many girls continue to function quite efficiently even when obviously debilitated. Anorexia nervosa is not catching in the usual sense but it can turn into a hysterical epidemic, especially in a girls' boarding school. If the genuine sufferer leaves, the rest of the so-called anorectics soon forget it. Headmistresses will use their own judgement. The older a girl is when it develops the less likely is she to be asked to leave, as her contemporaries are probably mature enough to understand her problems without being personally affected by them. Both O- and A-level examinations and degrees have been taken and successfully passed from psychiatric wards and anorexic units.

A girl's anorexia nervosa may be suspected by her school before her parents are aware of it. Her work may deteriorate, her handwriting or drawings alter, her meals may not be finished or even started, she may avoid her friends. The games staff are often the first to notice that a girl is losing weight or taking an unusual amount of exercise. They may notice that she feels the cold badly.

Headmistresses sometimes find that parents are reluctant to accept that their daughter may have anorexia nervosa, even after a talk with her or a letter from the school doctor. The parents cannot face the possibility of their daughter having to leave the school at an important stage in her education. They do not realise that the sooner they accept the anorexia nervosa the greater chance there is of a cure or even reversal and the less chance there is of their daughter having to be removed from the school.

Schools might find it helpful to use the biology lessons to explain the dangers of weight loss, the effects on the eyesight and reproductive system, the risk of other illnesses developing as a result of malnutrition, the psychological dangers of starvation.

Games staff could emphasise the undoubted benefits of physical fitness, of a properly balanced body, and particularly of the important function of good posture. There is a typical 'withdrawal' posture which characterises anorexia nervosa, shoulders bent, arms hanging slightly away from the body, chin poking forward. It has occasionally been found that this posture results from spinal malformation. It is not the result of anorexia nervosa but may have helped towards its development. Few schools now do remedial exercises for poor posture but no one can fail to feel better and more confident if they can face the world straight and upright. It is worth taking medical advice if a girl is standing badly in addition to any other manifestations of being unwell.

It is important that a girl continues to attend school regularly if possible, but her mother needs to make sure she is not getting over-tired. Doctors can be obsessed with a girl's undeniable need for autonomy and independence. They may need to make more allowance for the natural course of anorexia nervosa. Over-concern may intensify the illness but callousness does not help either. It is sensible for a mother to consider a doctor's insistence that a girl must go to and return from school alone. She should obviously do so when she has a stable acceptable weight, albeit on the low side, for her age and height. It is stupid and unkind to expect any girl to do so when she is very emaciated and clearly exhausted. She may be chronically fatigued, or she may take any available opportunity to run everywhere instead of walking. On both counts, it is realistic for the mother to take her daughter to and from school if she thinks it is necessary. She must use her own judgement, while remembering that the sooner her daughter can travel alone the better it will be for her.

It is a great pity that school teachers see supervising school meals as an unacceptable imposition. At one time they felt it was a natural part of their duties to see that their pupils ate regularly, knowing that a child who is properly fed is more likely to be able to concentrate and work effectively.

Cafeteria school meals and regular packed lunches are unhelpful. Not only is the real ritual importance of people eating together ignored but eating is reduced to the satisfaction of appetite. This does not acknowledge the importance of eating as a way of establishing and maintaining contact with other people. It makes it easy for a girl so inclined, to limit her intake of food to low-calorie foods at school. She can then go home and tell her mother what she knows she wants to hear – that she has eaten a large meal at lunchtime (often described in great detail). It is therefore quite unreasonable, she says, for her mother to expect her to swallow more than a few mouthfuls for supper. Unsupervised meals also enable girls who binge and vomit to eat far too much without either having to raid the larder or ask for or steal money from their mothers with which to buy extra food.

Other girls in a school may ask the headmistress or form mistress for advice. Anorexia nervosa has an unsettling effect and they may veer from over-concern to scorn when trying to help an anorectic friend. They may understandably try to force her to eat, they may be scathing and unkind. Neither helps.

The staff can help by explaining that anorexia nervosa is not an illness which is deliberately self-inflicted and that it may be reversed quite quickly or it may last for several years. Staff do not help by singling out the anorectic and giving her the extra praise and responsibility which they feel, often quite rightly, might help her. Other girls may easily resent any extra attention given to an anorectic although they are usually desperate to help her themselves.

A school can help enormously by explaining to the girls in an anorectic's form that the greatest help they can give is to never ask her to eat anything, to try to involve her in what is going on, to take her to their own homes without asking her to a meal, and of course to never, ever, refer to her physical appearance.

SIBLINGS

Most mothers are concerned and unhappy about the effect their anorectic daughter is having on her brothers and sisters. No one can live with an anorectic and remain unaffected; this shows itself in different ways. The mother undoubtedly has to bear a great deal of the blame for this since she could make life easier for the siblings if only she could keep quiet.

Not only are they subjected to terrible pressure by constant fights during mealtimes, during which they are naturally expected to continue quietly eating their own food, but they are in the unenviable position of being a captive audience. The mother's distress has only one real outlet – talking. Siblings may be subjected to endless and repetitive diatribes about their sister's behaviour but can usually say little in her defence, even if they wish to do so.

They are often just as worried as their parents about her declining health and emaciation, having a constant reminder of their own mortality. They may be embarrassed and frightened by mental illness and terrified that the same or worse will happen to them. They also, most worryingly in the case of younger children, have in front of them a spectacular example of the effectiveness of a hunger strike.

Siblings inevitably feel and often are neglected. The wild behaviour and alarming 'acting out' sometimes seen, particularly in younger siblings, represent a perfectly normal human need for warmth and contact. They are afraid to ask friends to come home because meals are a nightmare. A mother may give them the impression that they are being selfish in demanding the same amount of time and attention to which they were accustomed before their sister developed anorexia nervosa.

A girl with anorexia nervosa will not be helped by her siblings becoming increasingly estranged from her because they resent the concern and attention she receives. The illness never improves a girl's relationships with her siblings, with or without professional help. An anorectic often feels envious of and inadequate in comparison with her siblings – much to their surprise. She may feel guilty if she has always been preferred or given extra attention and presents by her extended family, possibly resulting from her difficult birth, being the only girl in a family or in some other way regarded as 'special'. Her insecurity and possible jealousy may lead her to see something sinister in almost anything her siblings say and do.

The mother needs to make sure that they are eating normally. This is difficult in a family in which conflict is expressed in terms of eating. The mother's control of her anorectic daughter's eating must extend to the rest of her family. They can indulge their scruples about eating dead animals, fresh vegetables, carbohydrate, eggs, milk and cheese when they are independent.

When there are small children in a family and the patient is at home all the time her mother may need to find some way of feeding the small child or children separately, while only cooking one meal. She can either feed them at different times, involving spending more time than she should over meals, or obtain the assistance of a friend, relation, nanny, or someone provided by the social services to eat lunch regularly with either the small child or the anorectic daughter. It is bad for small children to be continually upset by difficult atmospheres or appalling rows during meals. They may develop eating problems for which they cannot fairly be blamed. Seeing her siblings refusing to eat reinforces both the anorectic's feeling of control and her self-destructive guilt, adding to the vicious circle of eating difficulties.

A mother needs to maintain contact with the siblings, as it is easy to miss early-warning signs of disturbance. They need her time and support but she will not help them by making allowances for any bad behaviour or 'acting out'. They need to know that their mother is strong and determined, and that she is as concerned about them as she is about their sister.

The position of a girl with anorexia nervosa within her family affects siblings in different ways. When the eldest daughter develops anorexia nervosa it presents inescapable problems for a younger child or children. They have to enter adolescence hampered by family tensions and the extra support many of them give to their mother. They need considerable resources of courage and resilience not to flinch at the daunting tasks ahead of them. It is not surprising that some younger sisters become anorectic. Mothers sometimes feel that doctors regard the younger sister as copying the older one, rather than having problems of her own, and make little real effort to help her.

When the girl with anorexia nervosa is the second or subsequent child the older brothers or sisters may have reached the stage when they are beginning to leave home. Their departure is sometimes precipitated by the illness, the mother missing their companionship and help. Mothers have occasionally found that a determined attack on the anorexia nervosa by an older brother or sister prevents it developing.

If it is the youngest daughter who develops anorexia nervosa there can be additional problems. She may be alone at home with a mother who likes having her daughter with her, fearing a future without at least one of her children to look after and fuss over. A daughter who is afraid of growing up and who has no younger siblings pushing her forward may see no reason why she cannot stay a little girl for ever if her mother allows her to. Her mother may reinforce her helplessness by protecting her from her siblings. She may be able to use her involvement with her sick youngest child as a barrier between herself and a husband from whom she may have grown away. She may unconsciously cling to her youngest child so that her daughter becomes increasingly enmeshed with her mother, increasingly unable to separate herself from her mother, and eventually afraid of doing so.

A girl with strong and achieving siblings, either older or younger, may welcome the chance which anorexia nervosa gives her to withdraw from competition. In fact, even strong siblings usually feel that their anorectic sister has and has always had the upper hand.

It is essential to maintain or re-establish an anorectic in her position within her family. The mother can encourage the siblings to do this by doing so herself, making it clear that an older sister is still the older sister even though she is temporarily unable to assert herself. Both the sufferer and her siblings need to continue in their original roles within their family, and younger sisters will not be helped by their mother allowing or encouraging them to behave as though they are older than they are, under the illusion that this will help their sister.

Brothers can help by taking their sister with anorexia nervosa around with them, meeting their friends and being with boys or men as a matter of course. It may not be sensible for a brother to take too much responsibility for his anorectic sister as she may be seriously upset when he has a steady girl friend or gets married and so no longer has time for her.

A mother needs to avoid burdening the siblings emotionally. She needs to listen to their often sensible and relevant comments without over-reacting, listening to what they have to say and considering it calmly. A girl with anorexia nervosa may need reuniting with her siblings. The mother may find it possible to do this by providing them with a common enemy – herself. There is a lot to be said for losing her temper with them all at once, or making unreasonable demands or criticisms, until they go off together for some peace.

The mother must reinstate the boundaries within her family and not allow her children to make the rules. They need her to be in control so that they can get on with their own lives. She must not discuss her children with one another but must respect their confidences so that they can all trust her. She must be discreet and loyal to them all.

The mother must do everything she can to treat her

children the same, not making allowances or excuses for her anorectic daughter or giving her more of anything, not blaming the siblings for her illness or clinging to her daughter herself. She needs to maintain through thick and thin her attitude that anorexia nervosa is a difficult illness of uncertain duration which is making life awkward for them all at the moment but which can and will be cured.

Siblings may be afraid of having to look after and be responsible for a sister with chronic anorexia nervosa once their parents are dead or unable to care for her.

Anorexia nervosa which has lasted for more than seven years can and does become chronic. Improved knowledge and understanding, better treatment of the illness and earlier diagnosis should help to make this less frequent. A woman who is chronically anorectic may be able to live independently and often most successfully while remaining dominated by food and appetite and obsessively concerned with her weight and figure. She may be married and have children; she may have a dreadful existence, being totally isolated and constantly unwell.

Her mother may have decided long ago that she could no longer be responsible for her daughter. They may have lost touch or only meet occasionally. Nevertheless siblings know that when their parents die they will have to be partly or completely responsible for her welfare. They may have to support her or arrange for her to go into a home or hospital. They may feel morally responsible for her children, perhaps taking over where their own mother left off. It may be sensible for parents to make financial provision for a daughter who is chronically ill so at least that burden is removed from the siblings.

Siblings may be angry, resentful, neglected, guilty, impatient when their sister has anorexia nervosa. They are seldom sympathetic and find it hard to support a sister who rejects their offers of help. Their mother can do most to help by referring to the illness and its difficulties as seldom as possible. The less she says about it the less the siblings will be aware of it. The less they are aware of it the more help they will be to their sister and so indirectly to their mother. Both the mother and the father can learn from the Wise Old Owl: 'The more he heard, the less he spoke. The less he spoke, the more he heard.'

10

Hindsight

Oh, misery, my mother tears me down.
Stone upon stone I'd laid, towards a self
and stood like a small house, with day's expanse around
  it, even alone.
Now comes my mother, comes and tears me down.

She tears me down by coming and by looking.
That someone builds she does not see.
Right through my wall of stones she walks for me.
Oh, misery, my mother tears me down.

Rainer Maria Rilke

To conclude, here is some advice collected from other mothers and coloured from hindsight by my own experiences and observations. It does sound bossy but a mother who is full of self-doubt is not helped by having other doubts imposed upon her. I am reminded always of the mother who said to me that all the love and goodwill and care in the world are not enough unless they are supported by information and practical advice.

* Take medical advice as soon as you notice your daughter's weight loss and altered behaviour.
* Do not reject suggestions by other people, such as your GP or your daughter's school, that she may be in danger of developing anorexia nervosa. There is no reason to be ashamed of your daughter having anorexia nervosa. It does not mean that you are a bad mother, or that there is 'something funny' in your or your husband's family. She

may be seriously ill but she is not going mad. There is a popular misconception that anorexia nervosa leads to schizophrenia. This is *not* true.

* Be prepared to take a firm stand with your GP and do not hesitate to use your right to move to another practice if he is unwilling to keep a regular initial check on your daughter's lessening weight. There is nothing wrong with making a dreadful scene, if necessary in the waiting room, if this is the only way to persuade him to pay attention to her weight loss. He has a table of average weights relative to height, build and age. If your daughter's weight is less than 80 per cent of the average it merits attention. If she is of about average weight and maintaining it you may be worrying unnecessarily.

* Ignore any comments about her being at an age when her health is her own concern and none of your business. Anorexia nervosa is an illness which can and does have a damaging and even disastrous effect on the whole family. If she lives with you, and even if she does not, her health is very much your business.

* Try to be calm and polite for as long as possible but do not worry about being described as neurotic, hysterical, unreasonable and over-anxious. This is inevitable.

* Listen carefully to everything her doctor or consultant psychiatrist says to you about your daughter. If you feel he is wrong, try to discuss his comments calmly with him. Take with you at each visit a list of everything you want to know. Many mothers have difficulty remembering what has been said to them. If you have this problem take a tape recorder with you, either bought, borrowed or hired. This enables you to have an exact record of what was said and may encourage the doctor to restrict his comments to the relevant rather than to indulge in unnecessary speculation. It will also make it easier for you and your husband to discuss the doctor's views.

* Do not worry about being disloyal to your daughter. It is

essential to be completely honest and frank in your replies and in your description of your daughter's infancy, childhood and character as you perceive it. If she had difficulties with her peers or at school, or with any particular friend or member of your family, say so. If she took a fiendish delight in teasing the cat, say so. If she has an outstanding talent or ability, a need to care for others, a marvellous way with small children, talk about this too. If she is still mourning the death of a friend, parent or grandparent mention it. If she has had, or you think she has had, an unhappy sexual experience say so. Do not worry about any hidden meaning in a doctor's questions and do not feel on the defensive if these seem unkind or hostile.

* Sort out your priorities. If her doctor or hospital feel she is not well enough to cope with the undeniable pressure of examinations, please accept what you are told without feeling that all the hard-earned money, effort and time you have put into her education so far have been wasted. Her physical and mental health are too important to risk pushing her to the limits of both, possibly without success. She has the rest of her life in which to be educated.

* If your daughter's doctor feels that she should leave her boarding school and go to a local, perhaps less academically successful or well-regarded school so that she may live at home, please listen to him. Advice of this sort is not given lightly since no doctor and no reasonable school want to disrupt your daughter's education unless it is felt to be essential.

* Do not feel that her school must be at fault when the anorexia nervosa manifests and so take her away. This may be the beginning of a series of 'failures' which will make success and normality retreat further and further into the far distance.

* Do understand that if the illness is not appreciably or completely better within a year you are likely to be in for a

long haul. Make sure you are properly organised to with-stand several years of possible worry, fear and disruption, none of which will alter the illness for the better.

* Do not indulge in self-pity or panic. Buy a notebook and pencil so that you can work out rules and guidelines both for yourself and your family. These need to be flexible but firm.

* Make yourself a timetable, making sure that in doing so you do not set yourself impossible or over-demanding targets. It requires careful thought as once you have made it you must stick to it. It will help to clear your mind and help to counter the inevitable chaos which anorexia nervosa so often brings with it, so making the atmosphere calmer.

You need time in any one week to:

1. Do your domestic chores, cleaning, laundry, shopping, cooking, etc. Try to allow a set time for these as it is only too easy to droop about ineffectively for most of the day, ending in an exhausted panic, feeling guilty and depressed.

2. Spend time with your husband. He needs time to talk to you about his own concerns. Try to talk to one another, rather than at one another, and listen prop-erly. Your husband may alternate between rage and despair, feeling himself losing contact with this daugh-ter with whom he identifies. If you are strict with her he will feel you are unkind, if you are not then he will say that you are wet. He may be hurt by the way in which his anorectic daughter will tend to cling to her mother no matter what her underlying feelings may be. If he asks what he can do to help, suggest that he arranges something for you to do alone together, a long walk, a visit to the pub, the cinema, the theatre every week. The anorectic condition can exert a moral pressure which results in parents feeling guilty if they go out

together alone. Do not allow moral or emotional blackmail to make you give up any prearranged outing.

3. Take regular daily exercise out of doors. Walking is excellent, giving you time to think calmly. It will help you to sleep more soundly, if this is a problem. Worry makes people mentally rather than physically tired and regular exercise should help to counteract this.

4. Attend to your appearance. Your daughter's lack of self-confidence may relate to your own, which may evaporate, and you will feel much better if you know that you look nice. Many women find they put on unwelcome weight when their daughter has anorexia nervosa. This reflects both depression and the dietary chaos which often affects every member of an anorectic's family in some way. If you are alone make sure you have a nourishing meal at lunchtime rather than coffee and biscuits followed by more coffee and biscuits.

5. Be with each of your children individually doing something which they enjoy. They need you and you need the reassurance of seeing that you do not have the disastrous effect on them which you seem to have on your anorectic daughter.

6. Do something which you really enjoy, one afternoon or day each week. If you are working, try to organise one evening a week for yourself instead. Try to spend this time with other people who are not aware of your problems – do your best not to mention the anorexia nervosa. This is not selfish or self-indulgent. The distraction will help you to see everything more rationally and you will feel refreshed and stimulated which will help your family.

* Make sure you do all the family shopping and cooking. You may be able to prepare meals when your daughter is out, so lessening the amount of time you spend in the

kitchen when she is at home. Mothers know that often a daughter likes to sit and chat while a mother is cooking and they welcome the opportunity to talk to her. However when she has anorexia nervosa a mother needs to find some other time to be alone with her daughter – perhaps when she is sewing, watching television, listening to music, going for a walk.

* Remove all recipe books which are about diets and diet food. Do not buy magazines about health or slimming. Let her pay for them herself or do without. Do not be persuaded to buy any diet foods or aids.

* If she vomits you can lock the lavatory before meals. If she insists on being sick for several hours give her a plastic bowl and put her in the garden. Mothers have found that if a daughter continually vomits into bags which she then hides in her bedroom, under the mattress, in a wardrobe, in her shoes or Wellington boots, it is best to collect everything together every morning and put it in the middle of her bedroom, making it clear that she must dispose of it.

* If a girl is sick all over the table during a meal you will know that she is being aggressive because she is panic-stricken at her inability to refuse food. She wants to be told what to do. Give her the cloth, disinfectant and bucket and tell her to clear it up, making sure she cannot leave the room until she has done so. However distressed you are you must not clear it up yourself or pretend that it never happened.

* Ignore her exercising, providing it is not disturbing you or anyone else in your family. If she runs everywhere all the time tell her to stop it every time you see her – this sometimes works, on the principle of water dripping on a stone.

* Try to maintain some kind of physical contact with her, however minimal. There is a real benefit in being touched and in touching. If she leaps away from you when you touch her or washes the part of her skirt she thinks some-

one may have brushed against, she is not trying to tell you that you are dirty and disgusting, although it will feel like it to you. She is rejecting what you represent to her – authority, control, femaleness, sexuality – and which she temporarily wants to ignore.

* Try not to take personally her rejection of your food. Tell yourself that she is not rejecting your love and care or trying to humiliate or embarrass you. She is again rejecting what she sees of you in herself, especially the female attributes with which she is uncomfortable. She is fighting her dependence on you which she rightly feels is preventing her from achieving her own individuality.

* Restrict the number of times you allow yourself to launch into a tirade beginning 'What have I ever done to you to deserve this? All I ever wanted was to be a good and loving mother . . .'

* Never do anything for her which she can equally well do for herself.

* Having made a decision on any issue stick to it.

* Try not to hang around her. Your daughter needs faith, support, encouragement, firmness, fun. She needs her mother's loyalty and love but she does not need to have her mother constantly drooping round her bedroom door with a doleful expression.

* Try to organise things to do without feeling disappointed if they are not a success. On the other hand, try not to make allowances for behaviour which you would not otherwise tolerate. If she agrees to go out with you she should be ready on time or be left behind. If she decides to sit alone and miserable during an interval while you are all having a drink that is up to her. Allowing her to disrupt other people's lives and amusements will not do her any good.

* If she is frightened of a particular occasion discuss it with her. She may find it difficult to be in a social situation with her contemporaries knowing that they have been spending

the last few years widening their horizons while her energy and attention have been inexplicably concentrated on food. Do not allow her to use feeble excuses to avoid seeing her friends – the more she goes out and mixes the better she will feel.

* Do not discuss her with her friends. Do not try to prise information out of them about her behaviour with them or at school and particularly not about her eating habits. They will not tell you the truth and will eventually avoid coming to see her because they do not like being cross-examined by you.

* Do not ask your daughter's friends to try to make her eat. This is your responsibility and she needs her friends to talk to. It is not fair to burden them.

* She may be helped by talking to a friend's mother.

* Her friends come to see her because they like being with her, enjoy her company, know more than you think they do about the problems she has found within her family. They do not come to see her in order to give you an hour off from self-imposed martyrdom. Thanking them for being kind to her may humiliate your daughter and embarrass them.

* Do not flirt with her boy friends. Teenage girls feel much more secure if they see their mother as a grown-up woman rather than as a rival or twin sister. If your daughter sees you as her best friend, or if you do, it is high time she had another one.

* Try not to discuss her with her siblings or them with her. Allow each of your children to have their own relationships with you and your husband and with one another, knowing that they can trust you not to disclose their secrets to another.

* Never be afraid of precipitating a row. She needs to release her self-destructive anger. Avoiding arguments is only going to prolong her illness, although constant bickering and sniping are also damaging. Anorectics are

terrified of arguments but feel compelled to produce them.

* Any disagreements she has with her father or siblings are none of your business. If she is old enough to control her weight she is old enough to work out with whom she gets on. If you interfere you may only annoy everyone concerned without doing any good.

* Ignore as far as possible any minor aches or pains, maintaining the expectation that she is going to school or work as usual. By showing concern and rushing for either the telephone or the aspirin you are enabling her to use her illness as an escape. Try not to be frightened by the prospect of the serious illnesses which some anorectics develop. Resist trying to frighten her out of anorexia nervosa by telling her flatly that it is a well-known fact that all anorectics commit suicide, are unable to have children or develop stomach cancer. She will be as pointlessly upset by this as you are by your friends telling you about all the – quite different – cases they have heard about at third-hand who have either died agonising deaths or recovered splendidly in about two weeks.

* If she is constantly treated as ill she may relapse into perpetual invalidism and chronic anorexia nervosa. She is like someone recovering from flu, needing understanding that she is ill combined with the expectation that she is gradually getting better. She may sometimes be very depressed and will need encouragement and diversion.

* Recognise that her vulnerability may continue long after her weight has been restored. There is a *real* need to avoid contact with the supernatural and with quasi-religious groups like the Moonies. She needs the people she is with and the influences to which she is exposed to be as normal and as wholesome as possible.

* Try not to assume that everything that goes wrong with your marriage, her siblings, your motor car, the dog, the drains, the refrigerator or your management of your

housekeeping money is automatically her fault. There is a need to control an unbalanced reaction to all and every problem which enables you to use her as a scapegoat.

* Try not to look at her more than you have to. Anorectics are over-conscious of being looked at and observed all the time. If her skeletal appearance and frailty upset you too much you can always leave the room. This sort of attention is not good for her.

* As the illness progresses, she will find it harder and harder to communicate with you. You may feel that she bears no relation to the daughter you used to know and love and this may continue for a long time. Re-establishing contact as she emerges from a period of isolation and withdrawal requires considerable adjustment, as she will have changed and developed and so will you.

* It is essential to keep on talking, however hard this may seem. Even the most inane babble is better than brooding silences. She may be naturally disinclined to chatter and her withdrawal leads to almost total silence. Try not to take her withdrawal as a personal slight to you. Persevere with your efforts, remembering that she needs calming like a nervous kitten not working up into an emotional frenzy. Keep on trying to make contact with her without feeling hurt or rejected, because she is not psychologically or physically strong enough to respond to you.

* Her weight gain and general development will eventually help you to accept one another again.

* Reconnection is necessary. Do peaceful jobs such as sorting out photographs with her. Help to reinforce her sense of identity by talking about your and your husband's families and about her childhood. Get in touch with relations or friends with whom you have lost contact as this may also help her. If you feel she is seeking attention, because she cannot continue to develop without more than she has already had, give it to her without drama. You may find yourself considering the difficult concept of

retrospective loving – wondering whether an intense and prolonged display of maternal devotion can compensate for any lack she may have felt when she was younger. A compensation is accurately defined as something which does not quite compensate. Reconnecting has to be delicately and carefully done. Your daughter needs to keep a distance from you emotionally and physically which you can help her to maintain by not being hurt by it. You need to be less involved with her, too.

* Even anorectics who have been cured for years retain an unusually strong hold on the hearts and emotions of their mothers. Your daughter needs to realise that you have a life of your own quite apart from your function as her mother. Her recovery may be hindered by a continuing need of yours to have and keep her dependent – you are yourself dependent on her dependence.

* Try to remember how you felt at her age – shy, awkward, argumentative?

* Try to remember how you felt about your family, your mother and father, your siblings, your friends, your ability to cope with being grown-up. Do you see any patterns being repeated?

* Try not to feel your daughter will never again lead a normal life – she probably will if you let her.

WHAT ARE THE MOST IMPORTANT WAYS IN WHICH I CAN HELP MY DAUGHTER?

Don't allow her to use anorexia nervosa as an excuse to avoid joining school or family activities and don't yourself use it as a means of excluding her.

Don't go on diets with her, agreeing to lose 1lb for every 1lb she gains, and don't shop, cook, read slimming recipes with her.

Don't encourage her obsession with her body by suggesting, encouraging or paying for her to go to an exercise class or by buying her new leotards in which to exercise.

Don't use her anorexia nervosa to attract attention and sympathy for yourself.

Don't ever, please, allow yourself to retaliate by making unkind remarks about girls who do not menstruate not being 'real' women.

Don't focus too much of your attention on her by trying to protect her from her siblings.

Don't be jealous of the extra attention her father needs to give her.

Don't be infuriated, insulted or terrified by her obsessions. These will probably pass – although she may need professional help with them – if you can regard them as part of her illness and unpleasant for you all temporarily.

Don't compare her favourably or unfavourably with your friends' children.

Don't ask her to get better for your sake.

Don't criticise her friends or yours.

Don't tell her how lucky she is to be herself and not someone else.

Don't dwell on the sacrifices you have made for her.

Don't rescue her when she is in trouble, either with her school, job, friends or the police.

Don't allow her to droop about at home when she is quite well enough to find a job.

Don't criticise the job she finds.

Don't tell her boy friends that she has been, or is, anorectic, in the hope that this will make them especially considerate towards her. It is up to her to decide whether or not she tells anyone about the anorexia nervosa. When she does get married, *don't* assume that it will be a failure, *don't* always be available when she thinks she needs you, *don't* help her with domestic chores which you feel will exhaust her, and *don't* tell your son-in-law he is being unreasonable in expecting normal, regular meals.

216

Do make it clear that you are not ashamed or embarrassed by anorexia nervosa and that there is no reason for her to be so either.

Do encourage her and, more importantly, allow her to help herself.

Do be honest without being spiteful.

Do ignore any minor aches and pains without feeling guilty.

Do ask her for practical help rather than emotional support, but without going into paroxysms of gratitude if she does the washing-up.

Do allow her to lose her temper without being upset by it yourself.

Do make rigid rules about food and money and stick to them.

Do show her how old she is by treating her in the same way as you would a non-anorectic girl of her age.

Do talk to her about anything you can remember of her infancy and childhood – it will help her to know how much you love her and may also trigger off memories of anything frightening or nasty which may have seriously disturbed her without your being aware of it.

Do keep your view of her doctor, hospital or therapist to yourself, realising that hurtful comments which she repeats to you may have been taken out of context and distorted. Try not to ask her what she talks about when she is with anyone who is trying to help her.

Do assume she will get better eventually. Whether she does so or not may depend on how much you want her to.

Do remember always that she loves you and you love her but that love and possession are not the same.

Do love, accept and value her for herself.

I have studied the illness as much as a layman can. I have looked at it from different angles, considered the interpretations put on it by people who deal with it professionally and by those who do not, in the light of my own and other people's experiences. I have theorised, rationalised, agonised and analysed but I have not been able to get to the heart of the matter. Insight eludes me.

I started to write this book because I felt that it was needed. Nothing I have heard or seen or experienced has changed my mind. I have been helped, hindered, enlightened, enlarged, divorced, inspired, informed, criticised, amused, frightened, infuriated, loved, loathed, sustained, raised up and cast down.

Throughout it all my conviction has remained that the greatest barrier to an anorectic's recovery may often lie in the attitudes taken towards her mother and the consistent witholding from the mother of useful and helpful information. It is always easy to blame other people but a mother must be ultimately responsible for her children. How any mother comes to terms with all the years of illness, fear and isolation endured by her daughter with anorexia nervosa I still do not know.

References and Further Reading

The following references relate to comments and discussion within the content of the book and are given so that those interested may look them up. The page numbers refer to the text pages of this book.

p. 50   Jung, C. G. (1933). *Modern Man in Search of a Soul*. Routledge and Kegan Paul, London.

pp. 59, 97   Dally, P. and Gomez, J. with Isaacs, A. J. (1979). *Anorexia Nervosa*. William Heinemann Medical Books Ltd, London.

pp. 81, 83   Minuchin, S. (1977). *Families and Family Therapy*. Tavistock Publications Limited, London.

p. 109   Ryecroft, C. (1972). *A Critical Dictionary of Psychoanalysis*. Penguin Books, Harmondsworth.

p. 92, 98, 121 Bruch, H. (1976). *The Golden Cage. The Enigma of Anorexia Nervosa*. Routledge and Kegan Paul, London.

p. 138   John Donne, Letter to Sir Henry Goodyere, September 1608. Included in *Poetry and Prose* (1938), Thomas Nelson and Sons Ltd, London.

FURTHER READING

This selection is divided into titles directly related to

anorexia nervosa and those concerning prayer and positive thinking.

Bruch, H. (1976). *The Golden Cage: The Enigma of Anorexia Nervosa*. Routledge and Kegan Paul, London.

Crisp, A. H. (1980). *Anorexia Nervosa: Let Me Be*. Academic Press, London.

Dally, P. and Gomez, J. with Isaacs, A. J. (1979). *Anorexia Nervosa*. William Heinemann Medical Books Ltd, London.

MacLeod, S. (1981). *The Art of Starvation*. Virago Ltd, London.

Palmer, R. L. (1980) *Anorexia Nervosa: A Guide for Sufferers and Their Families*. Penguin Books, Harmondsworth.

BOOKS ON PRAYER AND POSITIVE THINKING

Enoch, D. (1983). *Healing the Hurt Mind*. Hodder and Stoughton, London.

Giles, M. E. (ed) (1983). *The Feminist Mystic and Other Essays on Women and Spirituality*. The Crossroad Publishing Co, New York.

Harris, T. A. (1973). *I'm OK – You're OK*. Pan Books, London.

Kelsey, M. T. (1973). *Healing and Christianity*. SCM Press, London.

Peale, N. V. (1963). *The Power of Positive Thinking*. Cedar Books/World Books International, Croydon.

Schumacher, E. G. (1978). *A Guide for the Perplexed*. Abacus Books, Sphere, London.

Tournier, P. (1966). *The Adventure of Living*. SCM Press, London.